A woman and her family can be healthier both emotionally and physically because of the practical advice, personal insight, and honesty of *Postpartum Survival Guide* by Dr. Dunnewold and Dr. Sanford.

> —Jane Honikman, Executive Director, Postpartum
> Support International, Co-founder, Postpartum
> Education for Parents

An excellent resource for expectant and new parents, *Postpartum Survival Guide* presents the gravely misunderstood, and often mistreated, postpartum adjustment period with sensitivity and compassion. It provides a wealth of precise information woven with practical, realistic advice, help, and direction for new mothers and their families in an easy step-by-step manner for a time when NOTHING seems to be easy.

> —Mary Ann Doerr, R.N., M.S.N., Director of
> Women's Health Services, St. Joseph Hospital,
> St. Louis, Missouri, and a mother of four children.

Postpartum Survival Guide is a clear, succinct, and practical explanation with interventions that are healthfully interwoven with true compassion, empathy, and support. I am impressed by the confrontation of the cultural/societal myth of "maternal bliss" which fuels a new mother's guilt and feelings of "something's wrong with me."

Recommended reading during pregnancy or as a handbook after delivery.

> —Tracy Rounds Brennan, M.S.W., President,
> Martha Rounds Slimnastics

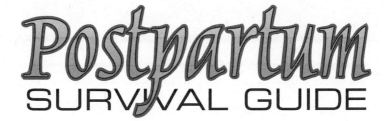

Postpartum
SURVIVAL GUIDE

ANN DUNNEWOLD, Ph.D.
DIANE G. SANFORD, Ph.D.

NEW HARBINGER PUBLICATIONS

Publisher's Note

This publication is designed to provide accurate and authoritative information in regard to the subject matter covered. It is sold with the understanding that the publisher is not engaged in rendering psychological, financial, legal, or other professional services. If expert assistance or counseling is needed, the services of a competent professional should be sought.

Copyright © New Harbinger Publications, Inc.
        5674 Shattuck Avenue
        Oakland, CA 94609

Cover design by SHELBY DESIGNS & ILLUSTRATES
Cover concept by Stephen Sanford and Shelby Tupper
Text design by Tracy Marie Powell

Distributed in the U.S.A. primarily by Publishers Group West; in Canada by Raincoast Books; in Great Britain by Airlift Book Company, Ltd.; in South Africa by Real Books, Ltd.; in Australia by Boobook; and in New Zealand by Tandem Press.

Library of Congress Catalog Number: 94-067045
ISBN 1-879237-80-6 Paperback
ISBN 1-879237-81-4 Hardcover

1st printing 1994, 6,000 copies

To my mother, Fran, and my daughters, Jessica and Rachel, who helped me learn about motherhood.

—Diane Goldstein Sanford, Ph.D.

To Randy, Abby, and Audrey.

—Ann L. Dunnewold, Ph.D.

Contents

Acknowledgments

As a mother who also works outside her home, I could not have succeeded in completing this book without the support of several people. First, I would like to thank my husband, Stephen. Whether it was taking our daughters out or doing an extra load of laundry, he made certain I had time to write. He listened patiently to my first draft, revisions, and editions. He encouraged me when my reserve was low.

My office assistant, Jane Talley, helped me with her enthusiasm, companionship, and public relations skills. Janet Karlen, my transcriptionist, was always available to lend her expertise. Our editor, Barbara Quick, dedicated her time and energy to this project in the midst of her new motherhood. My mentor, Dr. Arnold P. Goldstein, first read my scribbled outline for this manuscript and told me to get to it.

We would like to acknowledge Nancy Berchtold, founder of Depression After Delivery, and Jane Honikman, founder of Postpartum Support International. Without their commitment and vision, postpartum problems would still be hidden and ignored. Finally, we thank the women and families whose stories and lives have touched ours, and made this book possible.

—Diane Sanford, Ph.D.

I could not have written this book without the clients and their families who shared their lives with me. My deep gratitude and empathy go out to them in their struggles and their triumphs.

Many thanks to Diane Sanford, Marlene Joy, Dawn Gruen, Jane Honikman, Nancy Berchtold, Honey Watts, and Jeanne Watson Driscoll.

These women and many more members of Postpartum Support International and Depression After Delivery shared their ideas and insights, confirming that I was on track with my own. Without these people, I might still feel isolated and tentative in this world.

Thanks to Barbara Quick, our editor, and all the other helpful and receptive people at New Harbinger Publications, who made this book a reality.

Thanks to Mark Otis for teaching me years ago to trust my expertise and share it with others.

Special thanks to my parents, for instilling in me a belief in myself, and especially to my father for teaching me to write (with the help of Evelyn Roeder). I am extremely grateful to Phyllis and Darwin Payne, Solina Kasten-Marquis, and Callie Bower for their unwavering support and advice. And loving thanks to my husband Randy for always being steadfast and supportive, and to my daughters for their daily reminder of the joys and realities of motherhood.

—Ann L. Dunnewold, Ph.D.

1

You Are Not Alone, You Are Not to Blame, and You *Can* Feel Better

If you're reading this book, chances are that there's a postpartum crisis in your life. Whether it's your crisis, or a crisis being experienced by someone close to you, the first thing we'd like to tell you is to take heart! Things will get better. The postpartum period is an overwhelmingly difficult time—and anyone who tells you otherwise is lying.

There are measures that you and your family and friends can take to ease your stress, so that you can begin to enjoy your baby and feel like a human being again. Some of these measures may involve counseling and/or medication, depending on your situation. Other coping measures may simply be a matter of changing the way you think about things. Don't underestimate the power of your attitude and expectations. Changing the way you think just a little bit can make the difference between feeling totally out of control and feeling like you're under stress but coping.

Now, before we go on—if you're at the point where you're considering doing harm to yourself or someone else, you need to get professional attention right away. Call your OB/GYN, call a psychologist or social worker, call a suicide or child abuse hotline. You're going to be all right, and your baby will be all right, too—but you both need more help and support just now than can be found in a book.

How To Use This Book

This book is designed to be read in several ways. You may want to read straight through, or skip around, depending on your greatest need. Review the table of contents to see where you want to start. If you're still uncertain, read the summaries at the beginning of each chapter. Chapters 2 and 4 contain good introductory material. Begin with one of these, then read the other.

There is a lot of information in this book. Pace yourself. Read a little at a time. Move on when you're ready. You may want to reread parts of the book several times. In the usual state of fog of new motherhood, that may be necessary. Let your judgment of what you need guide you. Just keep plugging away, doing as much reading as you can manage at a time.

We know that one of your biggest problems is finding enough time to take care of your most basic needs: taking a shower, buying and preparing food, stealing a few moments to stuff it into your mouth (to say nothing of trying to get a few hours of uninterrupted sleep). Believe us— we've been there. Reading probably isn't very high on your list of priorities right now. If you're breastfeeding your baby, you might be able to squeeze some reading time into your nursing sessions. If you're lucky enough to have a baby who sleeps a lot—or you have a baby who nurses almost constantly—reading may already be part of your routine. To make the most efficient use of whatever reading time you do have, we've written a short summary at the beginning of each chapter. Read this if you don't have time for anything else. Each summary contains a suggestion for coping—either an easy-to-do exercise, or a behavioral or attitudinal change.

You might want to keep this book by the chair where you most often feed or nurse your baby. Read further as time allows; focus on the chapters that best fit your needs. Stick the book in the diaper bag when you go out. Look at a few more pages as you wait to see the pediatrician or your physician, or as you wait in line at the bank drive-through. Making time for reading this book is one of the first steps in the process of taking care of yourself. Setting aside ten minutes, morning or evening, and exploring the ideas contained here can be a great investment in *you.* If you take a little time to do something for yourself, you will find a payback in terms of more energy and better frame of mind.

Of course, if you've had the foresight to pick up this book while you're still pregnant—or if you're someone other than the postpartum mother—you can simply read this book straight through, from beginning to end.

All the books referred to in the text are listed with complete citations by category in the Resource Section.

Motherhood: The Hype, the Reality

Having a baby is supposed to mark one of the happiest times in your life. For nine months, you await your child's emergence with a whole range of emotions, from nervous anticipation to unadulterated joy. Society is quite clear about what your emotions are supposed to be once your baby is born. Television, movies, magazines, newspapers all give you the message that happiness, calm satisfaction, joy, and pride are the norm when a new baby arrives. Family, friends, and medical professionals tell you to "relax and enjoy your baby," as if relaxation played even the smallest role in the drama of life with a brand-new child.

Hardly anyone talks about the enormous physical, emotional, and relationship changes that accompany the birth of a new baby. Maybe it's because no one wants to be the killjoy sounding the notes of grim reality among all the soft-focus hype. But for many women and their families, the experience of having a baby turns out to be very different from their expectations. You may feel devastated when all your beautiful images of motherhood crash in a pile at your feet. "It wasn't supposed to be like this," you want to shake your fist and shout at someone. And the worst part of it is that no one wants to listen—not really. When you report that you're so sleep-deprived that you feel like an 80-year-old running a marathon, well-meaning friends and health professionals will tell you to sleep when your baby sleeps. Who do they think they're kidding? When their babies sleep, new mothers tend to their wounded bottoms, or throw some food in the oven, or agonize over the birth announcements they haven't even had time to buy, much less address the envelopes.

Your child may now be eight months old, or four years old, or having another child herself. This may be your first baby or your fifth baby. But in some way, you responded to the title of this book: what you are going through is different from what you expected.

The reality is that becoming a parent is a considerable task. The new mother's body appears to have gone haywire; her hormones fluctuate greatly. She is tired beyond belief, and suffering from sleep deprivation. Sleep deprivation, by the way, is a tried-and-true method for torturing prisoners of war! The new mother is in a physically vulnerable state from these changes and from the enormous physical stress of childbirth. And then, after a couple days' rest, if she's lucky, she is put in charge of meeting another human being's needs before tending to any of her own. Feed the baby, diaper the baby, rock or walk the baby, wash all the clothes that the baby has spit up on, and try to squeeze in your own shower, lunch, or fun. That is without even considering work, in or out of the home.

On top of these physical changes are emotional changes: you are now someone's mother, with all the psychological burden that role carries in our society. And having to put your child's needs first means that every other role you have played must be revised: partner, daughter, friend, worker. You may feel, quite naturally, exhausted, unsure, and overwhelmed. And because of the cultural myth of "this wonderful time," your negative feelings may have taken you completely by surprise. Since it wasn't supposed to be like this, you may find yourself feeling angry, cheated, and depressed. And who wouldn't, when you discover that the bliss and well-being you expected have been lost to feelings of depression, anxiety, and exhaustion?

What is most important to remember is that these negative feelings make sense when you look at the task a new mother is tackling. When you lack sleep, you are going to feel exhausted. When you take on a new job, it's normal to feel scared and uncertain. When you have little time to take care of your own needs for fun, companionship, and order, it's logical that you'd feel frustrated, resentful, and overwhelmed. Yet few sources of information for new mothers include a discussion of these negative feelings, or warn you about what to expect emotionally in the postpartum period. Instead, the myth of maternal bliss endures, leaving many women feeling cheated, depressed, and ashamed.

We need, as women, to replace this myth of maternal bliss with a more inclusive view of motherhood. You may have had an image in your head of baking bread and sewing baby clothes while your child slept in a bassinet by your side. Or you pictured yourself coming home to a smiling baby from your challenging and rewarding career each evening, full of energy and delight at your ability to "do it all." You and your partner would be closer than ever, the three of you a picture-perfect nuclear family.

Our new view of motherhood has to be more realistic and accurate. There are certainly tremendous rewards in being a mother, and these are not to be minimized or forgotten. But more emphasis needs to be placed on the challenges and difficulties that are part of the territory. Motherhood is not always the glowing and rewarding job it's made out to be. Being a mother is being in the trenches, mucking out the stalls, contributing much that is neither glorious nor immediately satisfying. Parenting is tough work. There are few absolute answers about how to do it correctly. And no matter how hard you try to do right by your child, you are absolutely guaranteed to make some mistakes. Society (not to mention those around the new mother) needs to support mothers more, validating the importance of the job. Good mothering is not only immensely valuable but essential to a healthy society. We need to recognize that mothers (and fathers) are fallible human beings. Many people have difficulty adjusting to their new job as a parent and all parents deserve society's support and gratitude.

We strongly feel that a more accurate idea of what you are getting into can go a long way toward relieving any guilt you may feel. If you know you're tackling a tough task, and others around you agree that it's a tough task and support you in your undertaking, you are less likely to feel badly if you stumble a bit along the way. If you expect something to be a breeze, and it turns out to be a hurricane, you may begin to doubt your aptitude as a parent, or to suspect that there's something wrong with you. Nothing could be further from the truth. Being a mother is demanding; if you find it to be so, you are completely normal. But you need the support of your partner, family, and friends in the process to keep your sanity and self-esteem.

We want to educate women and their families about the wide range of feelings that are possible after the birth of a baby. This book was written to let you know that having a baby is a tough adjustment: feeling lost or down or nervous is completely understandable.

The Wide Range of "Normal" Postpartum Adjustment

When you ask women what their postpartum adjustment period was like, you will hear a wide range of answers. Some new mothers feel wonderful, in charge, and confident. But many others report feeling rotten. Look at this list of feelings mentioned by women in a postpartum support group:

I am so irritable.	I cry all the time.
I can't sleep.	I can't get going.
I can't think straight.	I feel so worried.
I have panic attacks.	I can't stop eating.
I am nauseated.	I have scary thoughts.
I feel so nervous.	I feel so alone.
I feel so guilty.	I feel so ashamed.
I feel so ugly.	I feel so tired.
I feel like a failure.	I can't feel anything.
I have no interest in sex or other normal activities.	

We understand how difficult such feelings can be when you're faced with the myth that your life would be all rainbows. We know, as women and mothers first, and then as psychologists, the sense of guilt and failure when having that new baby in your life feels less than wonderful. In our work as psychologists, we've seen the relief in women's faces when their negative feelings are validated. Women feel crazy for having these feelings. They feel deficient and abnormal and ashamed. If it were possible to put a big motherly hug into words, this is what we'd do for every postpartum mom who picked up this book. In the words of Jane Honikman, founder of Postpartum Support International, we want you to know that **you are not alone, you are not to blame, and you can feel better!**

Why do we hear so little about postpartum emotions? Part of the answer is that society still wants to believe that new motherhood is nothing but wonderful. Women who have negative feelings in the postpartum period are afraid to talk: They feel as if something is wrong with them, that they'll be rejected by family or friends if they come clean about how they feel. They may not want to scare or worry other new mothers. This, combined with shame for their negative feelings, means that postpartum mothers don't even confide very much about their worst fears with other women. But a look at the statistics confirms how common postpartum reactions are. Researchers often find widely varied answers when they poll new mothers about their feelings. Generally, however, it appears that from 50 to 80 percent of all new mothers experience some short-lived negative feelings that can be classified as the "blues." And probably 10 to 20 percent of new mothers have a more long-lasting and more upsetting bout of negative feelings. There are no exact figures; but postpartum depression, anxiety, obsessive-compulsive, and panic reactions likely fall in this range, with 10 to 20 new mothers out of every 100 experiencing some of these difficulties. Finally, only 1 or 2 out of every 1,000 new mothers actually experience what is called postpartum psychosis.

A Guide To Feeling Better

Realizing that the feelings you have are neither unique nor your fault is only the first step toward feeling better. Our second goal is to give you some tools and strategies to use in managing your feelings and improving the quality of your postpartum life. In our work as psychologists, we've counseled several hundred women who were struggling with their feelings and behaviors after having a baby. From these women, we've learned a great deal about what works. Support is important. So is the knowledge that you are not alone, and are not the first person to feel this way. But you also need to take care of yourself. We agree with Ellen McGrath, Ph.D., chair of a national task force on women and depression for the American Psychological Association, and author of *When Feeling Bad Is Good*: she says that listening and talking are not enough. As Dr. McGrath prescribes, you must *act* for things to change.

The process of feeling better begins with letting go of self-blame. You can then tune into your own needs and the location of your anguish. What do you need most of all? How can you balance your own needs and the needs of those who are important to you, from the baby to other family members? What do your symptoms—the negative feelings or behaviors you have—tell you about issues you need to tackle? When you know what your needs are, you can begin to develop a plan to meet those needs. You can learn a new habit of taking care of yourself. We believe taking care of yourself to be critical to your physical and psychological health; it's also an essential skill in becoming a caring and successful parent.

Think of yourself as a pitcher of water. Every time you give to someone, meeting their needs, you are pouring water out of that pitcher. If you rock the baby, you are meeting her need for comfort. A little water pours out of your pitcher. You listen to your partner's report of a frustrating day. That takes a bit more from your pitcher. You take the baby for her checkup, draining the pitcher a bit more. You talk to a friend who had a big fight with her husband. By offering support, you are depleting your pitcher once again. The catch is that you are not a bottomless pitcher. You must stop at some point and do something to fill the pitcher up again. And how do you fill the pitcher? By taking care of yourself.

You can learn what works best to refill your pitcher. Some people like to relax in a hot bath, some people prefer exercise, or reading funny stories, or talking with supportive and nurturing friends. No matter what you do to fill the pitcher, it is essential that you do something. Otherwise, you will soon be empty. When you give and give without paying attention to your own needs, you're in danger of draining yourself dry. This book takes you through the steps of replenishment within the context of the extraordinary demands of new motherhood. We also provide concrete guidelines about when you need more help than you can provide for yourself, and how and where you can get such assistance.

About Breastfeeding

You may want to know about the effects of breastfeeding on your mood. This is a common question among overwhelmed new mothers. After all, breastfeeding involves firing up all those female hormones. Many women want to know if breastfeeding might be making them feel worse. They wonder if they would feel better if they quit breastfeeding.

The answer to that question must be evaluated on an individual basis. Some women do find that they feel much better when they are not solely responsible for providing their baby's food. Nonetheless, the research on postpartum emotional reactions very clearly shows that women who are breastfeeding do not have more negative moods than women who are bottle-feeding their infants. Instead, the hormones involved in the production and let-down of breastmilk often produce feelings of peacefulness and relaxation for the nursing mother. No matter what you may have heard to the contrary, breastfeeding does not mean that you'll have greater postpartum depression or anxiety. Nor does it put you at greater risk for feeling badly. In fact, if you are breastfeeding your baby and wean abruptly, you may find that your mood worsens because of the rapid change in hormone levels. Many women report increased negative feelings, such as depression and anxiety, when they wean their infants. So if you've recently weaned your baby, and were faced with an increase in your negative feelings or an unwanted change in your behavior, rest assured that this is not at all uncommon.

We've seen a disturbing trend in the treatment of postpartum reactions by medical professionals. Many of them appear all too hastily to prescribe antidepressant or anti-anxiety medications for the new mother who is feeling badly. Taking these medications usually requires abrupt weaning from the breast. Certainly, at times, this can be essential for the health of the new mom. But we feel strongly that, for women who are committed to breastfeeding, there are many other options to try *before* using medication. If breastfeeding is important to you, please know that you do not need to wean your baby, in many cases, if you do not really want to. You can first try the strategies outlined here before taking the more drastic step of weaning so that you can take medication. If your doctor seems cavalier in prescribing drugs, don't forget that you can always get a second opinion. Consult another physician, a lactation specialist, or a La Leche League counselor for support and advice.

To continue to breastfeed or not is your choice. You may need to "shop" to find medical professionals who will work with you to make your choice compatible with the help or treatment you need. We discuss this issue in greater detail in Chapter 7.

If you *are* feeling overwhelmed by the demands or difficulty of breastfeeding, you may wish to wean your baby so that you can share the responsibility for his or her nutrition. You may want to try a compromise solution rather than weaning the baby outright. Check with your pediatrician or a lactation consultant about supplementing your breast milk with formula. One or two bottles of formula a day (or during the night!) may give you the breaks you need, while allowing you to continue to nurse your baby. Too often, new mothers may see this issue as black or white (I must nurse exclusively/I need to quit nursing). No matter what anyone else says, there is a gray area in between (I can use formula to supplement and breastfeed, too). Many women who take an all-or-nothing approach and wean the baby because of their negative feelings in the postpartum period later regret having done so.

Women need to do what works best for them when it comes to breastfeeding. Do yourself the favor of getting as much information as you can and hearing both sides of the argument before you decide. It can be misleading to base your decisions on only one source of information, such as your child's pediatrician or La Leche League. There is no one right answer for everyone, because you and your baby and your particular situation are uniquely individual. Ask yourself what seems to work well for you and your baby. What doesn't seem to work? No authority in existence can improve on your own wisdom here. Books and health-care professionals can only provide guidelines about what has worked well for others in the past. Trust your instincts—this is the best advice anyone can give you.

If you truly feel that you are not enjoying breastfeeding and it is causing significant stress for you, you may want to wean your baby. Or you may feel that you truly need medication. Listen to what others have to say, but then make the decision for yourself. Don't listen to anyone who tries to challenge your decision once you've made it. (No matter what you decide to do, there is someone out there who will say that you made the wrong choice!) You need to trust that you know what is best for you and your baby. By remaining attuned to your needs, you can make decisions about your body that work for you.

Words of Encouragement and Hope

By now, you may be feeling some relief and hope that you can, in fact, get beyond this negative postpartum period. Facing up to the fact that this time in your life has not been what you expected is the first step. You may feel a lot of anxiety and uncertainty about whether you can succeed, for your life these days may feel like a failure. Listen carefully: you deserve credit for having the strength to tackle the difficulties of your life during this transitional time. Pat yourself on the back. You can do it. The fact that you've picked up this book and gotten this far is proof that you have the resources needed to make things better.

As you approach the task of feeling better, you need to keep your expectations realistic. In our clinical work, we've learned that the process of recovery is slow and difficult at times. It is always two steps forward, then one step back. You cannot take these suggestions and put them to work perfectly, with magical results. You are a human being, imperfect like everyone else, and cannot do everything you need to make yourself feel better every day. If you manage to persevere two days out of seven, then three days, and four, hooray for you! But if you expect every day to be good, you'll certainly be disappointed. There are always good days mixed with the bad, even under the best of circumstances. Just remember that the bad days don't mean that you've lost all your hard-won progress. When those days come, accept them as inevitable, and recognize them as survivable. Focus on the progress you're making. Keep in mind that you are not alone, you are not to blame, and you *will* get better.

2

Under the Rainbow:
The Spectrum of Postpartum
Adjustment Problems

The Short Version
(If You're Pressed for Time)

Even though you may have felt well-prepared for motherhood, some of your reactions may have come as a surprise to you. In this chapter, we describe the range of emotions that women often go through after the birth of a baby. You already know about the joy and delight a baby can bring. The rest of the story is presented here.

Because childbirth is a major life change, it's natural for you to have some negative feelings about it. The range of feelings different women may go through is much like the spectrum of light in a rainbow: the distinctions between the bands of color are not always clear; one color or category may blend into the next one. This chapter describes each level of negative postpartum reactions, from "the blues," which is the most common and least disruptive, to postpartum psychosis, affecting only 2 out of every 1,000 or so new mothers. We've provided checklists for each category to help you locate your own feelings along the continuum.

Until you have time to read our more in-depth descriptions and examples, here's the short course on postpartum depression and anxiety.

The Blues.   This is the term used to describe the common tearfulness, fatigue, insomnia, exhaustion, and irritability of the first two to three days after the birth of a baby. The blues are so common, striking 50 to 80 percent of all new mothers, that most health professionals pay little attention to the phenomenon. Feelings associated with the blues usually go away on their own within a week or two, and tend to be only slightly bothersome to the new mother.

Normal Adjustment.   The next level of distress felt by new mothers is categorized as "normal adjustment." "Normal crazy" might be a more accurate description. You may have many of the feelings of the blues, plus anxiety, mood swings, and anger. These feelings are completely normal, but feel crazy because of societal expectations that this should be a wonderful time in your life. In fact, these negative feelings of the normal adjustment period make perfect sense. New mothers are sleep-deprived, exhausted, and typically overwhelmed. They're thrown into a new job for which there's no adequate training available, and are given sole responsibility for a completely vulnerable and complex human being that arrives in the world without an instruction manual. The mother's negative feelings may continue for up to two months, and usually are "on again, off again" in nature, with many good days mixed in with the bad.

Postpartum Mood Reactions.   The collection of symptoms called postpartum mood reactions comprises the next step along the continuum. The new mother may be depressed, suffering from an amplified version of the crying, exhaustion, anger, mood swings, irritability, sleep problems, and self-doubt of the previous two categories. In the state called mania, she may have excessive energy, little need to sleep, and extreme irritability. Postpartum mood reactions last longer than either the blues or normal adjustment. The symptoms are much the same, but feel worse and interfere to a greater extent with getting daily tasks done. If you have many of the symptoms of the blues, and your baby is more than six weeks old, you may fit this category.

Postpartum Anxiety Reactions.   Like mood reactions, postpartum anxiety reactions involve an exaggeration of the negative feelings a woman may have in normal adjustment; but anxiety, worry, and panic are the primary symptoms rather than depression. Women who have anxiety reactions worry a great deal, have scary thoughts which they feel unable to control (this thought pattern is called obsessive-compulsive), or have panic attacks with many physical symptoms such as buzzing in the ears, tingling in hands or limbs, shortness of breath, dizziness, or flushed skin. Often these worries and panicky feelings are so troublesome that the new mother has difficulty getting her daily tasks done at all.

Postpartum Thought Reactions.   The rarest form of postpartum emotional reaction is a type of psychosis which occurs only once or twice among every 1,000 new mothers. In postpartum thought reactions, the new mother may have any of the problems described in the foregoing categories. But on top of these feelings and symptoms, she also has life-threatening confusion, hallucinations, or delusions that impede her normal functioning. Women with postpartum thought reactions see or hear things that are not there. They believe that what they are experiencing is real rather than illusory; as such, they can pose a great danger to themselves and their baby. Women with these symptoms need *immediate* medical attention.

Exercise:
Two Minutes for Yourself

You may find yourself being extremely self-critical, telling yourself such things as "You are so stupid! What's wrong with you that you can't even take care of your baby? You wanted this baby so badly and now all you can do is cry; get it together! What kind of a deviant person are you to have such terrible thoughts? What a lousy mother you are!"

Acknowledge what you are telling yourself; then imagine instead that you are talking to a child or a close friend who is tormenting herslf in this way. What can you tell her to make her feel better? How can you encourage her, and acknowledge all the hard work she's done so far?

Close your eyes, take four deep breaths, then say to yourself, "You are strong and competent, and this is really hard work. Just hang in there! Everything's going to be all right. Things will get easier soon." Draw on your compassionate side, and talk to yourself in the same gentle, supportive manner you'd use to cheer up a child or a friend who was in terrible pain. Do this for *yourself*. You are a special and wonderful person who deserves to be treated kindly.

2

Under the Rainbow:
The Spectrum of Postpartum
Adjustment Problems

Carol's Story

Like many young couples starting families, Carol and Paul had done everything in what seemed to be the right order. They finished college before getting married, and then launched their careers. They postponed having their first baby until they were settled in their first house. Down-payments and student loans behind them, Carol felt that she could take time from her career as a teacher to devote to full-time parenting. She and Paul embarked happily on trying to conceive a child, ecstatic that everything in their ideal timetable had gone so well up to this point. Month after month, as Carol got her period, their mood turned from happy to grim. But finally, after eight months, Carol surprised Paul at the door with a positive pregnancy test. They danced and shrieked, and began right away to plan the baby's nursery and study up on baby care and baby names.

The pregnancy went smoothly, and ended in a textbook labor and birth. Jenny was a healthy, easy baby, with a head of black tousled hair and blue eyes. Carol and Paul were in love with this sweet little being. Infant care took up lots of time, and Paul stayed home for the first week to trade baby-care duty with Carol. By the time Carol's mother arrived from her home three states away to help with the baby, the family seemed to be settling into a routine. All Jenny had done during the first week was eat, sleep, burp, and poop. Carol and Paul had enjoyed this first calm week, rocking the baby or gazing into her gorgeous blue eyes. Then something changed, and Carol was up three nights in a row with Jenny. The baby seemed to have her days and nights turned around, and would wail helplessly when Carol tried to lay her down in her crib. Carol's mother offered to take a turn rocking or walking the baby, but Carol wanted to do it on her own, despite her fatigue. This was *her* baby, and she wanted to be the first one to bond with her. She knew she would feel terribly inadequate if her mother could calm the baby down, when Carol was unable to do so. After those first sleepless nights, Carol broke down and cried uncontrollably five times in two days. Paul and her mother reassured her that this was probably normal—"just a touch of the blues." Carol was able to sneak in an hour's nap each of the next two days when her mother was there, and felt somewhat better.

The day when Carol's mom was scheduled to return to her own home, things fell apart. Carol was surprised to find herself crying and panicky at the thought of being alone with the baby. She had always considered herself to be a strong person. She had handled thirty 13-year-old kids in her classes at school. Why was she feeling so upset? Wasn't this what she had worked toward all these years? And here she was clinging to her mother like a 3-year-old left at preschool for the first time! This was the ideal she had been craving: a wonderful baby, a loving husband, and a comfortable home. And yet none of it felt right to her.

When Carol's mother left to catch her plane, she gave Carol a big hug. "You're strong, Carol—you'll find your way," she told her. But Carol found her mother's words hard to believe. The next weeks felt chaotic and unsatisfying to her. Everything was a blur of nursing, crying, snatches of sleep, and baby-oriented household tasks. As Carol became more and more exhausted, she started to worry, until she felt absolutely paralyzed by her worries. Could she do the right thing for the baby at any given time? Did Jenny want to be fed now? Or did she want to be rocked? Was she sleepy? Did her tummy hurt? The more Carol sought answers in her baby-care books, the more confused she became. She had difficulty returning to sleep after the baby's twice-nightly feedings, sometimes tossing and turning for three hours. She would seem to drift off just as the baby awakened again. When Jenny was five weeks old, Paul came home after his day at work to find Carol sobbing in the midst of piles of unwashed laundry and dirty dishes. He took the baby, tucked Carol into bed, and rubbed her back until she fell asleep.

At Carol's six-week postpartum checkup, she was obviously tired and withdrawn. Paul came home from work to stay with Jenny, sending Carol out the door for the doctor's office with the warning that she'd better tell the doctor what was going on. Carol's physician did question her about her adjustment to motherhood, but Carol answered mostly in monosyllables, giving only a sketchy picture of her sleeplessness and crying spells. The doctor patted her on the shoulder, explaining that she seemed to be having a rather bad case of the baby blues. He told her to nap when the baby napped, and get a sitter so that she could have a night out with Paul. Carol felt somewhat reassured, especially when the doctor told her she'd perk up when the baby began to sleep through the night.

Carol tried the doctor's suggestions for two weeks. Every day when Jenny fell asleep after her noon feeding, Carol laid down on the sofa to try and nap. She tossed and turned, just as she did at night. Paul arranged for the teenager next door to come over one evening so that he and Carol could have dinner at the new Chinese place just around the corner. They didn't get past the eggrolls before Carol was insisting they leave. She was too worried about Jenny, and wanted to go home and check on her *now*. Every evening after that, when Paul came home from work, Carol dissolved into tears. The tears might last all evening, or Carol might take a shower to calm herself down enough to eat some dinner.

One morning Carol became hysterical as Paul dressed to leave for work. She cried and ranted; she refused to be left alone. Both of them were surprised by her behavior—this certainly wasn't part of the lovely picture they'd envisioned. Paul called in to the office, and took the day off. He phoned every new parent and medical person he knew. Finally, he discovered a pamphlet on postpartum depression in the childbirth education packet they'd brought home from the hospital. The pamphlet listed the national self-help organization called Depression After Delivery. Paul called the toll-free number and received an information packet, a referral to a knowledgeable local psychologist, and the names of other parents he and Carol could contact by phone.

Normal Postpartum Adjustment and the Blues

Like Carol and Paul, most new parents don't expect a debilitating emotional reaction following the birth of their child. After all, having a baby is supposed to be one of the most wonderful times in a couple's life. Even when some difficulties are anticipated because of all the changes that accompany childbirth, the reality of postpartum depression is rarely considered. If it's considered at all, most prospective parents say to themselves, "That won't happen to me!"

Emotional reactions following the birth of a baby are often referred to as *postpartum depression*. You're probably familiar with the term. People use it for anything from constant tearfulness on the part of a new mom, to the rarer phenomenon of new mothers who have homicidal thoughts about their baby.

The more professionals have studied postpartum depression, the more they've concluded that it's not a single, distinct entity. Rather, a full range—or spectrum—of emotional reactions and symptoms appears to be possible in the postpartum period. These feelings and complaints most often take one of several definite patterns. This has led to the identification of related but varied emotional syndromes—or sets of symptoms—occurring after childbirth. *Postpartum depression, postpartum mania, postpartum panic reaction, postpartum obsessive-compulsive reaction, postpartum post-traumatic stress reaction*, and *postpartum psychosis* are the major patterns that we'll discuss in detail in this chapter.

To understand the range of difficulties women experience after the birth of a baby, the idea of a continuum is helpful. This is illustrated in the chart. The majority of new mothers undergo biological, social, and psychological changes that do not interfere with their day-to-day functioning, and are considered to be part of the normal adjustment to having a child. Approximately 80 percent of all women go through the *baby blues*, whose symptoms are listed in the left-hand column of the chart. The blues are a mild change in mood which occurs 24 to 48 hours postpartum, likely because of the dramatic hormonal changes brought about by labor and childbirth. Women with the blues report crying easily, reacting with irritation over trivialities they'd normally ignore, suffering fatigue, having difficulty sleeping, being more emotional than usual, or feeling slight anxiety or agitation. For most women, the baby blues do not last beyond two weeks, although some women may have mild symptoms for up to six weeks following delivery.

What is considered *normal postpartum adjustment* involves an extension of the symptoms of the blues through the first two months' postpartum. In other words, if you are past the timeframe for the blues, but still have many negative feelings, you've probably moved along the continuum into the normal adjustment category.

Normal adjustment is a misleading term, because you do not usually feel this way. Angela McBride, in her book *The Growth and Development of Mothers*, suggests that a better term would be "normal crazy." Most new mothers have maladjusted feelings and thoughts, but society leads us to believe that such reactions are somehow abnormal. In support of this view, the popular media portray new mothers as happy, loving, confident, and calm. This picture omits any negative reactions to the hard job of managing a new baby.

We believe that all new mothers experience some degree of "normal craziness" as they adjust to their new infant. The amount of difficulty a woman encounters depends on a host of biological, psychological, and social factors, and also on the type of baby she has (some babies are much easier to deal with than others). These factors vary from woman to woman, and for the same woman at different times in her life. It is rare for any woman to breeze through the physical adjustments and hard work of feeding, changing, and comforting a baby, 24 hours a day, all the while trying to restore her control over her own body. Most new mothers encounter periods of fatigue, depression, irritability, worry, tearfulness,

Spectrum of Postpartum Emotional Reactions

The Baby Blues	Normal Postpartum Adjustments	Postpartum Reactions	Postpartum Psychosis
☐ Crying	☐ Crying, tearfulness	*Depression:*	*Any symptoms from list at left, plus:*
☐ Irritability	☐ Irritability	☐ Worsening of normal adjustment symptoms	☐ Debilitating confusion
☐ Anger	☐ Anger	*Mania:*	☐ Hallucinations
☐ Insomnia	☐ Sleep disturbance	☐ Feeling speeded up	☐ Delusions
☐ Exhaustion	☐ Fatigue	☐ Decreased need to sleep	☐
☐ Tension	☐ Dysphoria (negative mood)	☐ Distractibility, pressured speech and thinking, irritability and excitability	
☐ Anxiety	☐ Appetite changes	*Panic reaction:*	
☐ Restlessness	☐ Loss of interest in usual activities	☐ Panic attacks	
☐ Emotionality	☐ Anxiety	☐ Extreme anxiety	
	☐ Emotional lability (mood swings)	☐ Physical symptoms—difficulty breathing, dizziness, shaking, etc.	
	☐ Feelings of doubt (re: attractiveness, parenting skills, etc.)	*Post-traumatic stress:*	
	Postpartum exhaustion:	☐ Panic attacks related to a specific past trauma	
	☐ Denial of depression or anxiety	*Obsessive-compulsive reaction:*	
	☐ Feeling overwhelmed	☐ Disturbing repetitive thoughts	
	☐ Inability to sleep or rest		
	☐ Physical symptoms (headaches, stomachaches)		

and doubts about their attractiveness and parenting skills. Mild sleeping problems, appetite changes, and a complete loss of sexual interest are also common.

Honey Watts, M.A., director of the Calgary Postpartum Support Society, has suggested that postpartum exhaustion may be a distinct category along this adjustment portion of the continuum. In postpartum exhaustion, women feel fairly well psychologically—they are neither depressed nor anxious. However, a woman with postpartum exhaustion may feel overwhelmed and "bone-tired," simply unable to function. She may not be sleeping well during the day or night. Instead of resting, she is busy meeting the needs of her baby, the household, and other family members. Mothers in this category may report numerous physical symptoms, such as headaches or stomach problems. The pattern of postpartum exhaustion is that many of these symptoms disappear when the baby begins to follow a regular schedule. As the baby starts to nap at regular times, and to sleep six or seven hours through the night, the mother can recover from sleep deprivation. This process can take several weeks, but then the new mother feels like herself again.

Many normal adjustment reactions are caused by the hormonal changes that accompany pregnancy and childbirth. But the enormous psychosocial transition of new motherhood must also be taken into account. When a woman has a new baby, particularly her first, she begins to reevaluate all her ideas about who she is. She may now compare herself, favorably or not, to her mother. She may have very distinct ideas about what kind of parent she wishes to be. She may wonder how she will put her former, childless self together with this new person who is suddenly a parent. If the new mother is changing her work status to care for the baby, these changes will be amplified.

Partners may face similar adjustments in self-image. New fathers must often deal with increased worries about financial needs and responsibilities. The demands on their time may mean that cherished leisure activities have to go out the window. They may be faced with a wife who isn't looking or acting at all like the woman they married. Plus they're expected to be involved with child-care responsibilities, even though many men have no model to follow in this area, as their own fathers were more than likely uninvolved.

The couple must also negotiate the mine field of their changed and changing relationship and household responsibilities. It's hard to make plans in advance when the baby's personality and the mother's condition after childbirth are a big unknown. All the ground rules for a household and a relationship change when a baby arrives. It's rare for a couple to simply know the right adjustments to make to find their sense of balance again.

New parents often need to reevaluate their relationship with the family in which they were raised. Becoming a parent may allow you a greater sense of adulthood and freedom from your family of origin. Or it may tighten bonds that have relaxed with time and distance.

With all these changes and negotiations going on, it's no wonder that the period following the birth of a baby is stressful. This is true whether the baby is the first or the fifth. With each child, the tasks, time demands, and alliances in the family shift. And, as with any stressful life stage, symptoms and negative feelings can easily manifest themselves. "Normal crazy" is usually not a problem. Most parents face it, and, with the support of family and friends, eventually regain some balance in their lives.

Things become more difficult if the new mother obsesses about what these reactions mean about her as a person. If she thinks her unhappiness or doubts reveal her to be a "bad," "sick," or less-than-perfect person, she may feel guilty. If she (or family members) question her mental health, parenting ability, or achievement of a bond with her baby, finding her balance again may be much more daunting. When these difficulties continue to affect her ability to get daily tasks done, or worsen over a two-to-five week period, a red flag goes up for a postpartum reaction.

This represents another step along the continuum of postpartum emotional reactions. Look at the foregoing chart again. It compares normal postpartum adjustment symptoms with the symptoms of postpartum emotional reactions. You may want to use this table as a checklist for evaluating your own symptoms. Place a check mark next to each problem you've experienced. If your baby is only one or two weeks old, your symptoms most likely fall into the category of the blues. If your baby is older than three weeks, review the symptoms in the normal adjustment category. Check those that apply to you now. If you have symptoms from this column, but they've persisted over two or three weeks, or have recently worsened, look at the next column under *Postpartum Reactions*. If you have symptoms in this category, you are likely having a postpartum reaction that needs attention. This is especially true if you are not getting up and dressed each day, or if you are not caring for your baby's needs.

In such situations, women cannot simply pull themselves up by their bootstraps: the situation needs to be dealt with immediately by a health-care professional who is knowledgeable about postpartum adjustment. If you think you're having a postpartum reaction, or someone you know is, use the resource list at the back of this book to find the best local people who can provide you with an evaluation and treatment plan.

Case Example: Normal Postpartum Adjustment

Liz was an associate in a high-powered New York law firm. Shortly before she was due to make partner, at the age of 41, she found herself pregnant. Both she and her husband were astonished, as Liz had never been pregnant before and always assumed she was just infertile. Her husband, another lawyer, agreed with her finally that they could give parenthood a try—but he made Liz promise him that she wouldn't let having a baby ruin her career. Their marriage had always been based on shared professional values and an attachment to the upscale lifestyle provided by their dual income.

Even though Liz got a lot of ribbing at work for "getting knocked up," the firm granted her an eight-week paid maternity leave. She continued working into her ninth month, and made it clear that she wanted nothing to do with a "mommy track" job—she still intended to make partner.

Then David was born. Liz fell in love with her baby more than she could ever have imagined possible. As her precious eight weeks at home with him began to whiz by, Liz became increasingly frantic. She kept telling herself that every moment with David had to count; she felt secretly worried that he wouldn't bond with her in their short time together. David was a placid baby and a good sleeper, but Liz found herself at the end of three weeks waking him up in the middle of the night so that she could nurse him and gaze into his eyes. She and her husband had gone to great pains to find a terrific professional nanny with impeccable references, but Liz tossed and turned at night worrying that they'd somehow made a bad choice. No one could love and care for her baby the way she did. She fantasized about handing in her resignation at work; she even fantasized about taking David and leaving her husband.

During the final two weeks, the nanny came to their apartment every day so that David could learn to be bottle-fed by her. Liz was supposed to spend this time resting or doing nice things for herself, but instead she locked herself in the bathroom and cried. How could she even contemplate returning to the cutthroat culture of the law firm with her leaking breasts and her sudden tendency to break into tears for no reason at all? How could she contemplate leaving David at home with the nanny? Liz's husband just shook his head when he came home one night and found her bedraggled, stained with breastmilk and spit-up, crying her eyes out. "Must be hormones," he said to her. "This just isn't like you at all. Remember, Lizzy? You're the one who makes other people cry!" Liz wanly nodded her head, making an effort to look cheerful for him.

During the seventh week, Liz switched moods like a traffic light changing colors. She sat for an hour, reveling in her baby's sweet gaze, rocking him as he cooed, feeling incredibly content. She wanted to soak up every tiny ounce of him, storing the feeling, smell, and sight of him to carry her through her return to work. Then she handed him to the nanny and ran from the room sobbing. Liz's husband brought her a new briefcase one evening to commemorate her upcoming return to work. She was delighted at first, then ended up raging at him for reminding her that her leave was ending. When the nanny gently suggested the next day that Liz might want to check in with her doctor before she returned to her job, Liz got furious at her, too, and then dissolved in tears. "I can't do this!" she wailed, relieved finally to be admitting the truth to someone. "I'm not even myself anymore. I don't know *who* I am! I used to be a very, very formidable attorney. Everyone was afraid of me."

"Of course they were," said the nanny, patting Liz's hand. "And they will be yet, as soon as your body settles down and finds its balance again. The best thing you can do for you *and* David is to get some sleep."

With help and encouragement from the nanny, who was really a very kind person, Liz managed to get herself together enough to make a decent impression when she returned to work. But she knew that becoming a mother had changed her forever. She still planned to make partner; but that long-sought goal had lost a lot of its meaning for her. She had a frank talk with her husband, letting him know that her values had really changed. Once she got her promotion, she planned to take a leave until David was ready for preschool. She had her whole life to be a highly paid attorney; but David would be a baby for only a very short time.

Postpartum Mood Reactions

Symptoms and complaints in the postpartum period that primarily involve changes in mood are categorized as a *postpartum mood reaction. Postpartum depression* and *postpartum mania* are the usual examples of these changes in mood or "affect." Research studies have shown that postpartum depression strikes from 10 to 20 percent of women with new babies. Figures are not available on the number of women who develop postpartum mania; but it's thought that mania may be a warning flag for postpartum psychosis, described later in this chapter. In very rare instances, postpartum depression can also develop into a psychosis. Postpartum psychosis only affects one or two in every thousand new mothers.

Postpartum Depression

The onset of postpartum depression is usually slow and gradual, occurring over a period of eight or more weeks. This mood reaction is characterized by it's on-again, off-again nature. A woman will feel great, then miserable, then good, then crummy, switching from high to low with surprising speed. This is distinct from the baby blues, which typically appear full-blown in the first few days after the baby's birth.

Postpartum depression can begin anytime during the first two months of your baby's life. The symptoms of depression are variable; but what distinguishes them from normal adjustment symptoms is that they persist after your baby is six to eight weeks old, and seem to affect you most of the time rather than just some of the time. You may notice extreme changes in appetite—either overeating or undereating. Changes in sleep patterns are also common—sleeping more, or having broken sleep.

Checklist of Symptoms for Depression

☐ Crying, tearfulness

☐ Irritability

☐ Anger

☐ Difficulty sleeping (especially returning to sleep)

☐ Fatigue, exhaustion

☐ Negative, depressed feelings

☐ Loss of intereset in activities usually enjoyed

☐ Anxiety and worry

☐ Quick mood changes

☐ Physical symptoms (i.e., headaches, stomachaches, muscle- or backaches)

☐ Changes in appetite or eating habits

Other symptoms include tearfulness and crying spells, a short attention span and problems concentrating, and spells of depression. A lack of energy and loss of interest in activities you usually enjoy are also characteristic. As with other hormone-related syndromes like PMS, you may find yourself increasingly irritable and overly sensitive.

Women with postpartum depression admit to feeling helpless and hopeless about their situation. They may fear particularly that they do not have it in them to be good mothers, or will be unable to ever care for their infants "in the right way." Many new mothers—like Liz in the previous example—fear that they have lost their familiar old self completely. You may begin to feel like a burden to your spouse, family, and friends, unable to redefine yourself in positive terms.

Faced with nagging self-doubts and negative feelings, a woman can rapidly lose her self-esteem. Many women who previously viewed themselves as competent and successful begin to see themselves in opposite terms—as failing and incompetent. Very often, this is accompanied by a tremendous sense of guilt about not living up to personal and social expectations about being a good mother. Women will say to themselves, "I just can't do this child any good," or "The baby deserves a better mother than I can ever be." As if this weren't enough, many women find their guilt compounded by worries about the effects of postpartum depression on the baby's development. Suicidal feelings, or thoughts about harming the baby, can haunt a woman as she struggles with these helpless, hopeless feelings.

To assess whether you may be suffering from postpartum depression, use the checklist of symptoms on the previous page. Read the list of symptoms carefully and think about which items apply to how you have been feeling. You may want to get input from someone close to you, such as your partner, another relative, or a close friend. It can be difficult to see your own situation clearly when you're right smack in the middle of it. Another person's perspective can help you get the "big picture," or may reveal a detail or pattern you just haven't noticed.

There's a good deal of overlap between normal adjustment and postpartum depression. As you read the following case example for postpartum depression, think about your own situation. The checklists and examples in this chapter won't provide you with an exact diagnosis—but they may give you an idea about the diagnostic category that fits you most closely. Based on this, you and people close to you can make a decision about whether or not to seek help from the outside.

Case Example: Postpartum Depression

Lydia was a 29-year-old mother of a robust baby girl. When the baby was five weeks old, Lydia found herself frequently crying when the baby cried. Helene was what the doctor called a "high-need baby," and cried a lot. There was plenty of opportunity for Lydia to fret. "What is the matter with me?" she wondered. "Babies are supposed to cry, and mothers are supposed to comfort them, not to join in." Before Helene's birth, Lydia had worked full-time as a psychologist. When her three-month maternity leave was up, she returned to work half-time, working three seven-hour days a week. Lydia knew only one other mother with an infant, and that friend worked full-time. There were no other people around on their street on the days when Lydia was at home. She felt lonely and isolated. To make things worse, all her friends at work were either unmarried or had children in college.

The days dragged on. Lydia brightened up when the baby had a few hours when her tummy wasn't hurting, when she was awake and playful. But when Helene started wailing again, Lydia couldn't stop crying. She felt like a complete failure as a mother, because she couldn't seem to do anything to comfort her baby.

Every evening Lydia badgered her husband to help find a solution. Had she made the wrong decision to bottle-feed Helene? Was there even such a thing as "colic," or was this just a meaningless, catchall term, as some experts said? Had Helene somehow been traumatized during the birth, or during Lydia's pregnancy? Had it been a mistake to have a baby at all? She felt like she was talking the issue to death. Her husband didn't say much when she talked, but gave her friendly pats, and murmured words of encouragement. Then one evening, at the end of an especially long discourse, Lydia's husband suggested that she really seemed to be overreacting. "We have a babysitter two days a week, and someone comes in to clean the house. Can't you just cope, Lydia?" he asked her. "After all, you're a psychologist—you know all about coping!" At this, Lydia just blew up! How could he be so calm, so smug, when her life was in such turmoil? She raged at him: *she* couldn't come and go as she please, *she* couldn't get a decent night's sleep! Her body didn't feel like her own—she couldn't fit into any of her old clothes. She didn't have a moment she could claim for herself. She was either at work, trying to look convincing as someone who could help solve other people's problems, or she was at home with a screaming baby who arched her back and wailed when Lydia tried to comfort her.

With some tears, talk, and hugs, Lydia was able to open up to her husband about how her life had changed, particularly in terms of her reliance on friends for support. Before the baby, her friends and confidantes had been psychologists like herself, childless and carefree. Now, these same friends looked bored when she talked about Helene's bouts of colic. More and more friends seemed to become mysteriously busy when she stopped by their desk for a chat. She even overheard one colleague in the restroom say to another, "Poor Lydia! She's completely obsessed with that baby. I can't find anything to say to her."

The next day, Lydia headed to the library, Helene in tow, to look up postpartum depression. Articles were scarce, but Lydia found more and more symptoms that matched her situation: she cried frequently, felt lonely and angry at times, and had even lain awake several nights worrying about her life. She realized that she needed to make some changes. There just didn't seem to be anything she could do about Helene's colic but wait it out; but she needed to find some other people who were in the same boat as she was.

After calling her doctor, the hospital, and her childbirth educator, Lydia discovered a postpartum exercise class, and was able to arrange with Helene's babysitter to cover the extra three hours a week. Lydia enrolled right away. The contact with other new mothers was great, as was the feeling that she was getting her body back.

Through the class, she met another new mother in her neighborhood who also had a high-strung baby, born just a month before Helene. Between the two of them, they managed to discover two other local mothers, and formed a play group. By the time Helene was three months old, Lydia felt much more at ease with her life, and had two important new friends. She could pick up the phone whenever she needed to make contact. And Helene's colic was easing off to the point where she only cried one or two hours a day, giving Lydia the chance to see what a lovely, lovable baby she really had.

Important Note

If you think you may be suffering from postpartum depression, you'll find guidelines for feeling better in the chapters on self-help (chapter 4) and professional treatment (chapter 7). If you feel there are symptoms you have struggled with that have not been addressed above, carry on with this chapter until your symptoms have been accurately described.

Postpartum Mania

Postpartum mania is likely to appear in the same time period as the blues, in the days immediately following your baby's birth. In postpartum mania, women frequently describe themselves as feeling "speeded up"; they have trouble relaxing or slowing down. They may have a decreased need for sleep. The woman with mania may sleep for only two or three hours a night, without feeling tired. Thinking tends to flow quickly from one topic to another. Listeners may have difficulty following the new mother's logic as she talks. Her speech patterns seem different from usual, with a rapid flow of words.

In mania, you may sound or feel under pressure to "get it all said." It sometimes seems like you're thinking faster than you can talk. The speed and excitability of your speech require a lot of energy, both to produce and to follow. Distractability is common in mania, as are instantaneous mood swings, for instance from excitability to irritability to depression. A woman in mania may seem to be a whirlwind of energy: she might make lots of lists of things to do, or clean house excessively, or undertake any number of difficult projects. However, these activities often turn out to be unproductive, as she jumps around from one task to another, leaving a wake of chaos behind her.

Unlike mania unrelated to childbirth, postpartum mania does not seem to be characterized by an elated or euphoric mood. What you'll mostly see is an increase in irritability or excitability. In the first week or so of postpartum mania, no one may notice an impairment in your thinking: faulty reasoning, poor judgment, and distorted perceptions may be at a minimum. But postpartum mania can progress to the level of such impairment very swiftly. If you're having symptoms like the ones described above, you should be treated by a competent professional as soon as possible.

To evaluate whether your symptoms fit the description of postpartum mania, study the checklist on the next page. Mark those symptoms that you've noticed in yourself since your baby was born. We'd encourage you to ask someone close to you to for their perspective on the situation. It can be difficult to see things clearly from inside your own head. The following case example may also be of use to you in determining whether you might be suffering from postpartum mania.

Case Example: Postpartum Mania

The early days after the birth of her first daughter were a nightmare for Nancy, a 36-year-old, stay-at-home mom. Nancy hardly rested at all between her daughter's nursing sessions every three hours, sleeping only a couple of hours a night. Instead of feeling tired, she described herself as "bursting with energy." She rushed around the house trying to get things done, but accomplished little as she flitted from one task to another. She would fold laundry for two minutes, then get out the vacuum cleaner, leaving it in the middle of the hall while she went off to scrub the bathtub. When her husband John came home one night, there was wet laundry on the couch, and rice burning in a pot on the stove. Nancy was out in the driveway starting to wash the car. The baby was asleep in her swing.

Nancy made long lists of what she had to do, but didn't seem to have the attention span needed to finish any one task. The lists kept getting longer and longer. She spent much of her time each day talking on the phone, even talking at length to telephone solicitors. After a couple of weeks, John, friends, and other family members noticed that Nancy's conversations weren't making much sense. She couldn't keep her mind on any one thing; she kept tripping over her words in her urgency to get everything said. Nancy was frequently irritable, and would snap at her husband for such trivialities as bringing home the wrong brand of milk. He began to dread coming home.

Alarmed by these changes in her behavior, Nancy and John finally consulted a psychiatrist. Nancy was put on *Lithium*, which meant that she had to wean Anna earlier than she'd planned. But, gradually, Nancy's symptoms subsided. There was no discussion at the time of postpartum mania or continuing psychotherapy, and for years the couple struggled to understand why Nancy had acted so strangely. Nancy was extremely concerned that something similar might happen if she had another child.

When she became pregnant again, Nancy had to work up her nerve to inform her new OB about her history, fearing the doctor's negative judgment of her. John came along for support. After listening quietly and respectfully, the doctor said that Nancy seemed to be suffering from guilt

---

Checklist of Symptoms for Mania

- ☐ Feeling "speeded up"
- ☐ Little need to sleep or rest
- ☐ Distractability (thoughts jump quickly from topic to topic)
- ☐ Speech seems very fast, pressured—tripping over words
- ☐ Irritability
- ☐ Easily excited, especially susceptible to anger or disappointment

about how crazy she had acted when Anna was born. He suggested that Nancy consult a psychologist who specialized in postpartum difficulties.

Nancy had difficulty at first opening up and telling her whole story to the psychologist. She was afraid that her behavior would be held against her; that she might be seen as an "unfit" parent. John came along again, at Nancy's request; and he had no qualms about revealing all the details. The psychologist was not the least bit shocked, as Nancy had expected her to be, but simply set out to educate and reassure Nancy and John. They learned that Nancy had experienced postpartum mania, triggered primarily by hormonal changes following childbirth. Armed with this understanding, Nancy slowly accepted that her odd behavior hadn't been her fault. She realized with relief that she wasn't a bad mom, as she had labeled herself, but simply a woman who had survived a serious postpartum reaction.

Important Note

If you feel that your own symptoms match our description of postpartum mania, you can find guidelines for feeling better in the chapters on self-care and professional help. If your symptoms have not yet been clearly described, please read the next sections below.

Postpartum Anxiety Reactions

Postpartum depression and mania primarily involve changes in your mood levels. Postpartum anxiety reactions consist of heightened and recurrent feelings of anxiety and/or panic. The anxiety and worry can be vague and nonspecific, focused on life and the world in general; or they can be related to specific events and situations. Fears and anxiety-provoking thoughts about the baby are characteristic. Clinical varieties of postpartum anxiety reactions include *postpartum panic reaction*, *postpartum obsessive-compulsive reaction*, and *postpartum post-traumatic stress reaction*. These are described in some detail below.

Specific figures are not yet available on the numbers of women experiencing these reactions, which have only recently been identified by researchers. The estimate of 10 to 20 percent, cited above for postpartum depression, probably includes a lot of anxiety reactions, as there's some overlap between the two diagnostic categories. Anxiety symptoms usually manifest themselves in the first two to three weeks after the birth of a baby, but may not reach a distressing level until several weeks later. If symptoms are not identified and treated promptly, a woman may become depressed in reaction to her anxious feelings. The typical new mother expects to feel confident and happy after her baby is born, and may wonder if there is something gravely wrong with her for having such painful worries. Self-doubt and guilt over not being able to control the worry can only worsen the natural blue feelings—the normal crazy—of the postpartum period. This can throw the new mother into considerable depression as well.

Postpartum Panic Reaction

Women with postpartum panic reaction frequently remark that their panic attacks and anxious feelings "come out of the blue." A panic attack is an episode of extreme anxiety in which a person experiences physical symptoms that may include

- Shortness of breath
- Chest pain or discomfort
- Choking or smothering sensations
- Dizziness
- Tingling in hands or feet
- Trembling and shaking
- Sweating
- Faintness
- Hot and cold flashes

People who are in the throes of a panic attack may fear that they're dying, going crazy, or losing control. A general sense of restlessness, agitation, or irritability may be present. All of these symptoms can be continuous or off-and-on. If you have panic attacks, you may have difficulty identifying a particular event or situation as the trigger. The lack of a provoking incident leaves many women feeling even more helpless and overwhelmed.

It's common for people having a panic attack to believe they're actually having a heart attack, and to seek medical attention. When no circulatory problems are found, medical personnel must rule out digestive difficulties (such as heartburn or esophogeal reflux) or systemic illnesses (such as *lupus erythematosus*).

Some postpartum women have panic attacks a few times a week, while others may have attacks almost continuously each day. It's even possible—and quite common—to be awakened from sleep by these symptoms.

No matter how frequently you get panic attacks, you never get used to them. Having a panic attack is a truly agonizing experience. The dreadfulness and intensity of the symptoms can leave you exhausted, vulnerable, and apprehensive about the symptoms returning.

Some women with postpartum panic reaction also have recurrent fears and thoughts about harm coming to their children, other loved ones, or themselves. The new mother may get stuck on these thoughts. Such obsessive fears can make problems with depression or anxiety even worse.

You'll probably recognize whether your symptoms fit the description of postpartum panic reaction. It may also help you to refer to the list below. Read through the checklist of symptoms carefully, marking those you've had since your baby was born. Read the case example that follows for further perspective on your own situation.

Case Example: Postpartum Panic Reaction

Mae was the 24-year-old mother of a 6-month-old boy. Her symptoms began with the blues—she cried nonstop from the day her son was born. Mae was afraid to take care of the baby initially. She had little experience with infants, and at just under six pounds, the baby looked so tiny and fragile. Mae showed so little confidence handling the baby that her husband George was worried. He called his mother, who agreed to come stay with them for several weeks.

George's mother was a matter-of-fact sort of person, and took on the task of teaching Mae how to care for her baby in a concrete but gentle manner. By the end of her mother-in-law's three-week stay, Mae had "gotten her feet wet," and felt fairly confident about handling the baby on her own.

Then George was laid off from his job when baby Eric was only two months old. As they tried to recover from this blow, Mae and George planned a long weekend trip together. Eric still wasn't sleeping through the night. Mae and George thought they'd combine a much-needed break

---

Checklist of Symptoms for Postpartum Panic Reaction

- ☐ Extreme anxiety
- ☐ No specific event seems to be a direct cause of anxiety
- ☐ Shortness of breath
- ☐ Chest pains or discomfort
- ☐ Choking or smothering feelings
- ☐ Dizziness
- ☐ Tingling in hands or feet
- ☐ Trembling and shaking
- ☐ Sweating
- ☐ Faintness
- ☐ Hot and/or cold flashes
- ☐ Fear of dying, going crazy, losing control
- ☐ General restlessness and agitation
- ☐ Extreme irritability

from parenthood with a job-hunting trip to a nearby city. George's mom came back to care for the baby.

Mae had some dizziness and nausea before leaving on their trip, but chalked this up to a virus. She wasn't about to sacrifice their weekend for some mild flu symptoms. While stopping at a cousin's house on the way, Mae suddenly felt overcome by the heat, even though the weather was mild. Her face, arms, and chest felt on fire. She was having difficulty getting her breath, and felt as if everyone was drifting away from her. George took her to the hospital, while Mae gasped, "I'm going to die," over and over again. Her blood pressure and EKG were fine, and the emergency room physician gave her a prescription for *Xanax*, an anti-anxiety medication. Mae refused to believe that the intense feelings she'd had were "only anxiety." When she returned home, she was given a thorough battery of tests by her own doctor, who somewhat hesitantly diagnosed her as having lupus, an inflammation of the connective tissue. The doctor admitted to Mae that the blood tests were inconclusive, but he prescribed high-blood-pressure medication, and Mae continued on the *Xanax*. Her panic attacks continued undiagnosed for several more weeks, with Mae feeling intense hot flashes, chest pains, and horrible fears that she was dying. Still unenlightened, her doctor gave her nitroglycerine for her chest pains. Mae was devastated, certain that she'd die young, leaving her baby son without a mother.

Then one day in the doctor's waiting room, Mae discovered an article on panic attacks in a magazine. She realized that her symptoms fit the description perfectly. The stresses of her husband's loss of his job, and their separation from the baby during the weekend, had triggered the initial panic attack. Mae consulted a psychologist, who helped her talk for the first time about her parents' divorce when she was seven, which was haunting her still. With the psychologist's help, Mae learned techniques for handling the panic attacks without medication, and for coping with stress in general.

Important Note

If you feel that your postpartum symptoms have now been clearly described, you can find guidelines for feeling better in the chapters on self-care and professional help. If not, continue reading below.

Postpartum Obsessive-Compulsive Reaction

In postpartum obsessive-compulsive reaction, the primary symptom is the recurrence of persistent and disturbing thoughts, ideas, or images. These arise spontaneously, without intentional thought, in the first couple of weeks of postpartum. Most commonly, these spontaneous and disturbing ideas have to do with harming your baby somehow. Prevalent fantasies include hurting the baby with knives, or putting the baby in the microwave oven. Other women have reported thinking about suffocating their children, throwing them down stairs, or drowning them. Women who are survivors of childhood sexual abuse may have thoughts or fantasies of molesting their children in similar ways. Other loved ones—such as an older child, a partner, or a parent—may be the object of these fantasies. The possible harm imagined can include accidental events, such as automobile crashes, or such illnesses as cancer.

Thoughts like these are actually common in new mothers as they become acutely aware of how vulnerable babies are. Evelyn Bassoff, Ph.D., in *Parents Magazine* (October 1993), says that imagining such trauma befalling your baby is a common response to hearing about violence in the world. You may play out these disturbing ideas over and over in your head in an effort to make sense of them. This may be a way to feel more in control and ultimately better able to protect your child in a dangerous world.

Obsessive thoughts, nonetheless, may cause a woman a great deal of distress and self-loathing as she again asks herself, "What is the matter with me for thinking this way?" Unlike women who develop postpartum thought reactions and cannot separate fantasy from reality, women with obsessive-compulsive reaction are quite aware that their thoughts aren't real. They are thoroughly repulsed by their images, and rarely experience the urge to act upon them.

If these symptoms seem to match your own experience, you probably feel terrible about the thoughts you've been having. They don't at all reflect your true feelings—you don't want to harm your child. Far from it: your child is the most precious thing to you in the world.

Your destructive images may be the result of feelings you haven't allowed into your conscious awareness. Negative feelings that don't fit with a woman's expectations for parenthood may come out indirectly in this manner. If you expect parenthood always to be fun and rewarding— rather than tiring, draining, and frustrating at times—you may become disillusioned with the experience of having a new baby. Anger at your situation, your spouse, or other family members can result. You may be so invested in having everything turn out *right* that you can't let yourself acknowledge your angry feelings. But feelings have a way of making themselves felt, whether or not you suppress them; and in the process they can become quite distorted.

A less frequent symptom of postpartum obsessive-compulsive reaction is the performance of ritualistic behaviors to protect yourself from having bad thoughts. Women may hide the knives or avoid the kitchen in an effort to ward off thoughts of harming the baby with knives. Some women may avoid basic care, refusing to bathe their baby out of fear of their thoughts about death by drowning.

There are many variations on these types of thoughts and related behaviors; we've only given a small sampling here. But if our descriptions seem to fit with your own experience, take a look at the checklist that follows, and mark those symptoms that sound familiar. Understanding that your thoughts are just thoughts, and that you aren't likely to act on them, may enable you to ignore them sufficiently to go on with your day when they arise. Professional treatment, including medication, is needed if you are not able to dismiss these thoughts for what they are—ideas in your head. Women with postpartum obsessive-compulsive reaction are *always* clear that such thoughts are both wrong and offensive, and that they shouldn't be acted on.

The differences between postpartum obsessive-compulsive reaction and postpartum thought reaction or psychosis, described later in this chapter, are 1) the knowledge that the thoughts are wrong and should not be acted on, and 2) the disgust the woman feels in reaction to her thoughts of doing harm. Women with postpartum obsessive-compulsive reaction have not been known to carry out their disturbing thoughts, while women with postpartum thought reaction are not repulsed by their thoughts and may actually put them into action.

Case Example: Postpartum Obsessive-Compulsive Reaction

Carolyn was a 38-year-old mother of a son. Happy to be home from her bank job caring for her sweet, sleepy baby, she was shocked when she began to have thoughts of hurting him. When the baby was one week old, the idea of putting him in the dishwasher just "popped into her head" as she loaded the dishes. This was followed by thoughts of putting the baby in the oven. The thoughts then progressed to a vague, "I could so easily kill him."

The thoughts terrified Carolyn. She felt she had turned into a monster. How could a normal person have such thoughts at all? She tried closing her eyes and squeezing her temples to stop the thoughts. She played loud music on the radio all day to drown them out. Neighbors in her apartment complex complained to the manager. When she couldn't

---

Checklist of Symptoms for Obsessive-Compulsive Reaction

☐ Repetitive, persistent thoughts, ideas, images

☐ Such thoughts arising "out of the blue"

☐ Having thoughts that are disturbing or alarming

☐ Having thoughts about harming your baby or other loved ones

☐ Clear understanding that it would be bad and wrong to act on these thoughts

☐ Feeling that you can't control these thoughts that keep coming into your head

play loud music anymore, Carolyn took the baby down to a local construction site, hoping the sound of the machinery would keep the thoughts from coming. But then she found herself fantasizing about losing control of the baby's stroller, of it rolling into the jaws of the backhoe.

By the third week, Carolyn was so scared that she might act on her thoughts, which she seemed unable to control, that she returned to work before her leave was over, and started volunteering for lots of overtime. That way her husband had to pick the baby up at day care, feed and bathe him before Carolyn even arrived home. She waited two more weeks before telling her husband about the thoughts, feeling tremendous guilt during that time. She would wake in the middle of the night, her heart racing with fear that the thoughts would overwhelm her and she would be driven to act upon them. Her husband was speechless at her revelation. He just picked up the baby and walked out of the room, leaving Carolyn sitting in a daze. But then he returned after a couple of minutes, and they talked.

Carolyn's husband encouraged her to consult her OB, who prescribed an anti-anxiety drug, *Buspar*. This helped somewhat; the thoughts lessened. But Carolyn remained worried about whether she might still act on her thoughts. The OB had not explained anything about why such violent and hateful ideas popped into her head.

Carolyn continued to feel guilty and inadequate. She became depressed, and began to call in sick every day, staying at home while the baby was at day care. Her supervisor called one day to check on her, and encouraged Carolyn to call her OB again. She did, telling him about her feelings of depression and worthlessness, and her trouble getting going in the morning. When, in consultation with a psychiatrist, Carolyn's doctor prescribed an antidepressant medication as well, the thoughts disappeared entirely. Carolyn slowly resumed care of her baby, with lots of help and support from her husband.

Important Note

If you feel that your total postpartum experience has now been described, you can find guidelines for feeling better in the chapters on self-care and professional help. If you have symptoms that have not yet been described, please read on.

Postpartum Post-Traumatic Stress Reaction

Besides being a mouthful to pronounce, postpartum post-traumatic stress reaction describes another set of anxiety-related symptoms which may occur following childbirth. Perhaps you've heard or read about the syndrome called post-traumatic stress disorder, or PTSD. PTSD has come to the attention of the general public through news stories about soldiers returning to civilian life haunted by a range of painful psychological symptoms, from flashbacks to nightmares in which they relive the trauma of war. Rape victims, victims of other violent assaults, and people victimized by natural disasters such as hurricanes or floods are also subject to PTSD. The syndrome is similar, although not identical, in postpartum women.

As you'll recall from the last section, postpartum panic reaction usually has no clearcut triggers that set off a new mother's panic attacks. They just seem to come out of the blue. In postpartum post-traumatic stress reaction, the event that sets off the panic attack tends to be associated with a specific trauma—either a recent one, such as potentially life-threatening complications during labor and delivery; or a trauma from the woman's past. A past trauma can include any violent assault that you suffered as a child, or any accident in which you almost died. A new mother exposed to a situation that reminds her of this trauma is vulnerable to panic attacks—especially if she's had panic attacks before, although this is by no means always the case. Women in the throes of such an attack may fear that they'll die in the course of being subjected to the traumatic event a second time. For women who have had traumatic first births, attending childbirth education classes with their second pregnancy can remind them of the horrible experience they had, and set off a panic attack. Avoidance of the feared situation may occur; women who fear choking may stop eating solid foods out of fear of reexperiencing their earlier trauma.

Unlike some victims of violence who suffer from PTSD, most postpartum women do not have flashbacks in which they lose their grip on reality and actually believe themselves to be in the traumatic situation again. Nightmares about the trauma are also less common in postpartum post-traumatic stress reaction, although both flashbacks and nightmares are possible. Likewise, the numbing or emotional detachment in which the person can't feel anything related to the event is lacking in the postpartum version, even though it's common in post-traumatic stress reaction occurring with other life events. As with postpartum panic reaction, panic attacks or avoidance behaviors may wax and wane. Careful discussion and attention to the events surrounding each attack typically reveal a particular situation that provoked the reaction. This, again, is what differentiates the post-traumatic stress reaction from postpartum panic reaction, in which panic attacks appear to come out of the blue.

Clearly, at this point in the continuum of postpartum reactions, you would be well-advised to consult a knowledgeable helping professional about coping strategies and the possible usefulness of medication. To help you assess whether you are suffering from post-traumatic stress reaction, we've designed the checklist on the next page. Carefully study the list of symptoms, marking those that you've experienced. You may wish to ask your partner, another family member, or a knowledgeable helping professional to go over the checklist with you. Exchanging ideas with someone else often provides a clearer picture of your frame of mind. The case history that follows may also help you understand the symptoms in the context of a real-life situation.

Case Example: Postpartum Post-Traumatic Stress Reaction

Patti's pregnancy had been smooth and problem-free. Her problems started after 21 hours of labor, when the baby's heart rate dropped drastically, and the doctor performed an emergency C-section. She was emotionally and physically drained after her surgery, and didn't feel well enough to go home after the three days in the hospital covered by her insurance company. But Patti was someone who always expected a lot of herself, so she and the baby went home long before Patti felt recovered. As if this were not enough stress, Patti awakened in a pool of blood at 4 a.m. three days later. Her husband called a neighbor to stay with the baby, and an ambulance to take Patti to the hospital. The bleeding was so bad that both Patti and her husband were afraid that Patti was going to die.

It turned out that a major artery had been nicked during Patti's Caesarean. The doctors were able to repair it, but Patti was very frightened about leaving the hospital, and slept badly after she returned home. But her anxiety didn't escalate into panic attacks until Patti found herself several hours away from any major medical facility one Saturday, three months postpartum, when she and her husband were taking the baby to visit a relative in a rural, somewhat isolated part of their state. Driving down a bumpy, two-lane country road, through fields and woods, Patti began worrying that she might start bleeding again. What if she couldn't find competent medical help quickly enough? What if she died? They were out in the middle of nowhere. There were no comforting "Hospital—next exit" signs anywhere along the road; there weren't even any telephones! Patti's thoughts intensified into a panic attack, and she was swept up in the terror of her last hospitalization. She felt the same dizzying, breathless anxiety she had felt on the ambulance ride the night she had hemorrhaged.

Checklist of Symptoms for Post-Traumatic Stress Reaction

☐ Panic attacks in response to specific situations (see panic checklist on page 31 for symptoms)

☐ Previous trauma, either recent or long ago

☐ Sensation of returning to the traumatic event—illusion of actually being there

☐ Nightmares about the traumatic event

☐ Emotional numbness—inability to feel anything

After this experience, Patti stopped traveling anywhere she judged to be an unsafe distance from a major hospital. Thoughts about the horror she had endured, almost dying, overwhelmed her, and she continued to have panic attacks. When Patti returned to work from her maternity leave, she discovered that her job description had been expanded to include travel to remote parts of the state. Her immediate impulse was to quit, but she was afraid of what might happen if she lost her health insurance. She and her husband couldn't manage on one income, especially with the added expense of a baby.

With these challenges facing her, Patti consulted a psychiatrist about her panic attacks. She was fortunate to find someone who was both knowledgeable and sensitive, and together they explored the pent-up feelings and memories that had haunted her. Eventually, her panic attacks were brought under control.

Important Note

If you feel that your symptoms have now been correctly described, you can find guidelines for feeling better in the chapters on self-care and professional help. If some of your postpartum experiences still haven't been covered, continue reading in the sections below.

Postpartum Thought Reaction

Postpartum thought reaction is the term used to describe the extreme reaches of the continuum of postpartum emotional difficulties. As the term implies, a new mother suffering from this reaction has difficulties with her thought processes. This is not the mere forgetfulness or spaciness that's so common to postpartum women, but actually a form of temporary psychosis, wherein the new mother loses touch with reality. Changes in mood may or may not accompany the problems with thinking. Symptoms of postpartum thought reaction can range from moderate to severe, and can progress quite rapidly. The milder symptoms are extreme distractability and racing thoughts, as in postpartum mania. Significant confusion, poor judgment, and delusions or hallucinations may also be present. A woman might forget what task she is working on midstream. She might leave the baby unattended in a potentially dangerous situation, or completely misjudge the baby's needs. She may think, in a paranoid manner, that friends or family members dislike her, when in fact they are being supportive.

Complete loss of contact with reality—as in postpartum psychosis—represents the far end of the spectrum of thought reactions. Postpartum psychosis is the rarest of the postpartum emotional reactions, with only one or two new mothers in one thousand exhibiting psychotic symptoms. The onset of postpartum psychosis is usually early, within the first 24-72 hours after the baby's birth. But it can also occur at later times, particularly in conjunction with such physical stresses as abrupt weaning or severe sleep deprivation.

A thought reaction can last several days to several weeks, particularly if left untreated. It may begin with the new mother feeling a great deal of confusion, and expressing strange ideas that do not match with reality. It can progress to vivid hallucinations, further confusion, disorientation, and delusions about the baby. Postpartum hallucinations and delusions often have a religious quality. For example, a woman may believe that her baby is a demon who will harm her. Or she may believe that her baby is Jesus, or hear voices telling her that she's the mother of God. The severity and bizarre nature of these thoughts are part of what differentiates them from the obsessions that make up postpartum obsessive-compulsive reaction. The latter are related to more commonplace, day-to-day activities. Also—and this is crucial—women with postpartum obsessive-compulsive reaction have not been known to act on their thoughts about committing violence against the baby, whereas a woman in psychosis might.

Women with other postpartum reactions may have vivid fears and strange fantasies about their infant's health and well-being, but they can differentiate between these fantasies and reality. Women with postpartum psychosis accept their bizarre thoughts and beliefs as perfectly real. They may hear, taste, see, smell, and feel things that no one else can perceive. They can't be "talked out of" their perceptions, because they aren't thinking accurately or correctly. Because they're unable to distinguish fact from fantasy, these women may lose their ability to control the impulse to act on a thought, however violent or bizarre.

We've made a checklist of symptoms for a postpartum thought reaction, on the following page, just as we did for the other postpartum syndromes. But a person in psychosis is beyond the stage where self-diagnosis is useful or even possible. If you're close to someone you suspect may be suffering a thought reaction, read the checklist and mark those items that you think may apply. Whether or not the diagnosis is an exact fit, it's essential to get professional help right away. The lives of both the baby and the mother may be in danger. Use the resource list at the back of this book to find local agencies and helping professionals.

Case Example: Postpartum Thought Reaction

Elaine was someone who liked to do things right. She had an easy pregnancy, a "textbook perfect" labor, and a good early adjustment to her baby. At 36, she was delighted to become a mother, and her husband was ecstatic with their little daughter. Both grandmothers lived nearby, and took turns coming for the day to help out just after the baby was born. Elaine napped and read for two or three hours each afternoon for the first week, while one or the other grandmother took over with the baby and cooked dinner.

Elaine felt very confident initially, despite some problems with breastfeeding. By the end of the week, when both grandmothers decided to go back to their own busy lives, baby Amy seemed to have caught on about nursing. But that's when the bottom fell out for Elaine.

She hadn't fully realized how important all the help and support had been to her, always having someone there to take the baby, or to give Elaine a pat on the shoulder or encouraging words. She became depressed on her own, and was often so nervous that she couldn't accomplish much of anything during the day; at night she had tremendous difficulty sleeping. After Amy's two-week check-up, the doctor put her on a two-hour, round-the-clock feeding schedule, as she still hadn't regained the weight she had lost when nursing had been problematic. Elaine would lie awake watching the clock, afraid of missing a feeding, remembering the pediatrician's disapproving scowls at the last visit when the baby was weighed.

Elaine's husband had a job that required him to work twelve hours a day. Elaine just couldn't ask him for help when he arrived home looking haggard and exhausted at night. She herself was only sleeping two or three hours a night, and felt anxious and jittery much of the time. Her OB prescribed an anti-depressant medication that made it necessary for

---

Checklist of Symptoms for Thought Reactions

☐ Extreme distractibility—losing train of thought or forgetting what you're doing

☐ Thoughts jumping from one topic to another

☐ Extreme confusion—inability to accomplish simple tasks

☐ Poor judgement or decision-making

☐ Difficulty seeing or understanding things as others do

☐ Inability to distinguish fantasy from reality

☐ Hallucinations—seeing and hearing what isn't there

☐ Delusions—ideas that don't match reality

☐ Disorientation—inability to recognize familiar people or places

☐ Impulsive actions

☐ Sudden, irrational-seeming changes in mood

☐ Sleep disturbance—inability to sleep, or to fall back asleep after waking

Elaine to wean Amy long before she had planned to—which was a bitter disappointment after all the hard work of that first week. Elaine became even more of a nervous wreck, as her hormones jockeyed for balance again.

Like many babies, Amy fussed and cried every evening for about two hours. Elaine felt that she ought to be able to figure out what was "wrong," to give Amy what she needed. When the crying persisted, Elaine became increasingly frantic. She felt badly about taking the medication, believing that her recovery ought to be a question of "will." Didn't other women pull themselves up by their bootstraps as they adjusted to a new baby? Elaine's self-esteem was crushed as she replayed this question in her head all day and often all night. She truly felt she could do it, if she just worked hard enough.

Then, when Amy was almost three weeks old, Elaine and her husband had a huge argument about Elaine's inability to adjust, and her husband's procrastination about helping around the house. They called each other names and slammed some doors: each was certain things would improve if the other would just "get it together." They had never had such a big fight before. Elaine was terrified that it meant their marriage was over.

After the fight, Elaine couldn't sleep for four days running. Her depression and anxiety mushroomed, and she began to imagine ways to commit suicide. She felt she would rather die than lose her family to divorce.

After her fourth sleepless night, Elaine lost touch with reality. In a monotone voice, she reported to her husband that she had committed suicide, died, and was currently in Hell attempting to get to Heaven. She was completely withdrawn; her husband couldn't get Elaine to look at either him or the baby. She just sat on the bed with her arms wrapped around her shoulders, rocking herself and mumbling. As the day went on, and her husband made arrangements to hospitalize her, she became catatonic, unresponsive to anyone and unable to move her body at all.

Elaine entered a psychiatric hospital, was given antipsychotic medications, and was herself again in five days, although severely shaken by her experience. She continued outpatient psychotherapy after she was released, to address her perfectionism. She and her husband entered couples' therapy to deal with the marital distress that had triggered their fight.

Important Note

The occurrence of a postpartum psychosis is potentially life-threatening to both mother and baby, and requires prompt and aggressive medical attention. Women who have a personal or family history of manic-depressive illness are significantly at risk for developing postpartum psychosis. These women should be monitored by a mental health professional during pregnancy and following the birth of their baby. They also should be given as much support, household help, and supplemental care as the family budget will allow.

Beyond Diagnosis

All women experience some changes in mood and behavior as part of the normal adjustment to the birth of a baby. Biological changes, including dramatic hormonal adjustments, make it all the more difficult for a woman to struggle for emotional balance again as she gets used to being a mother and having a baby. This process is a major life event, and requires reevaluating everything about your social patterns and self-image.

Sorting out the difficulties and symptoms of the blues, normal postpartum adjustment, and postpartum emotional reactions can be quite a task. Keep in mind that symptoms of a postpartum emotional reaction are more extreme than the changes of normal adjustment, and generally worsen over time, especially if left untreated. The list that follows summarizes the most dangerous symptoms and stresses to watch for.

Eheart and Martel suggest in their book, *The Fourth Trimester*, that it's best to view uncomfortable feelings, such as those described here, as signals about your situation. Categorizing your symptoms can help you develop a plan to feel better, either on your own or in consultation with a qualified professional. It is not intended that you categorize yourself as a way of *judging* yourself. Rather, try to listen to what your feelings are telling you about your physical, social, or emotional state.

We've described each syndrome as if it existed in some distinct pattern along a continuum. But in real life, there is a lot of overlap between each diagnostic category. You may have symptoms of more than one reaction, or may move through the spectrum at different stages of your postpartum adjustment. Symptoms can begin during pregnancy also, and especially deserve attention then. If you or someone you know is exhibiting the behaviors described here that are beyond the range of normal adjustment, thorough evaluation and prompt intervention by a competent health-care specialist is mandatory.

The next chapter will help you to determine what extent you're at risk for a serious postpartum adjustment problem.

Danger Signs in the Postpartum Period

- Sleep problems that increase, especially problems returning to sleep after feeding the baby
- Eating problems—eating too much or too little
- An increase in depression or irritability, especially
  - Self-deprecating thoughts or self-doubt
  - Increasing discomfort with being a mother
  - Fears for the child, infanticidal fantasies
  - Death wish, suicidal thoughts
- Lack of steps to counteract fatigue (i.e., not napping)
- Avoiding people, becoming withdrawn, socially isolated
- Difficulty interacting with the baby
- Panic attacks
- Inability to reason; hallucinations, delusions
- Mania—feeling speedy, a decreased need to sleep, being distractable, irritable, excitable, and exhibiting pressured speech

3

Am I at Risk?: Biological, Psychological, and Relationship Risk Factors

The Short Version
(If You're Pressed for Time)

You may be afraid that you're having postpartum adjustment problems because something is wrong with you as a person. Rest assured that there's nothing wrong with you in particular—but it's easy for the physical and emotional stresses of childbirth to cause imbalances in the body, and your relationships.

For all women, having a child results in enormous biological, psychological, and what we're calling relationship changes. Under the best of circumstances, you're bound to feel tired and at times overwhelmed and uncertain. It may seem as if your world is falling apart. For almost all new parents, it seems as if the world has turned upside down.

Fortunately, a great deal is now known about the factors that contribute to postpartum adjustment problems. In this chapter we delve into the three main categories of causes: those which are biological, those which are psychological, and those which have to do with relationships. A risk profile questionnaire is provided to help you determine which factors may have contributed to your postpartum difficulties.

We've broken down each category into individual problems of symptoms, which we then describe in detail. The items in the risk profile questionnaire follow the same order, so that you can refer back to the explanations in the chapter if you're unsure about what is meant by an item on the questionnaire.

Until you have time to read our more in-depth descriptions of these factors, and to fill out your risk profile questionnaire, here's the short course on the causes of postpartum reactions.

Biological Causes

Biological causes include:

- Normal physical changes of pregnancy and childbirth
- Hormonal changes of pregnancy and childbirth
- Heredity
- A previous episode of postpartum reaction
- Complications of pregnancy and childbirth
- Breastfeeding and weaning
- Premenstrual Syndrome (PMS) and menstrual problems
- Thyroid imbalance

From what is currently known, if you have experienced a prior postpartum reaction, you have a 50 percent chance of having another one. With regard to heredity, your odds of experiencing a postpartum episode may greatly increase if your mother or another close female relative had a postpartum reaction, or if there's a history of manic-depressive illness in your family. Information about how strongly other biological factors contribute to postpartum problems is less clear, and may vary considerably from woman to woman.

Psychological Causes

Psychological causes include:

- Normal psychological changes accompanying childbirth
- Expectations about motherhood
- Lifestyle patterns
- Previous psychological problems

- Childhood experiences
- Unresolved losses
- Recent stressful life events
- Personal resources for self-care and coping

Experts suggest that up to 70 percent of all women who experience a postpartum reaction have no history of psychological problems. So even if there aren't many psychological factors contributing to your postpartum difficulties, the normal emotional upheaval accompanying childbirth is in itself a risk factor.

A woman's expectations about what her life will be like after having a baby, and what sort of mother she'll be, are of enormous importance to the ease or difficulty of her postpartum adjustment. The more perfection you expect, the more emotional trouble you're likely to experience when you come face to face with the realities of having a baby. Unresolved issues from the past may also complicate your adjustment, particularly if they bothered you just prior to or during your pregnancy. Having a child may cause unresolved issues from the past to surface. Stressful events that occur closely before or after the birth of your child seem to be a larger contributor to postpartum adjustment problems than stressful events from the more distant past.

Relationship Causes

Relationship causes include:

- Normal relationship changes following childbirth
- The quality of your marriage or partnership
- The quality of your social support system
- Being a single mom
- The quality of your relationship with your baby
- Your relationship with your other children

With constant demands on your time and energy, having a new baby can strain even the best of marriages. If relationship problems predate your child's birth, your risk of a postpartum reaction is greatly increased. The weaker your network of close friends and family to lend emotional support and assist you with child care, the more susceptible you'll be to problems after the baby's birth. Although less is definitively known about other relationship factors, the quality of your relationships is crucial to an easy postpartum adjustment.

Exercise
Two Minutes for Yourself

Try to remember a day in your life when you felt happy, peaceful, and self-confident. It doesn't matter if the memory is a recent one or from very long ago. If you don't have an actual memory to draw on, try to imagine what such a day would be like. Are there people around you or are you alone? Are you at the beach, in an office, on a stage, in a restaurant, or snuggled up in bed? Picture as vividly as possible the details of your surroundings. Use all five senses—identify sounds, smells, tastes, textures, and colors. Now pay attention to how your body feels on this wonderful day. What is your breathing like? Can you feel your heartbeat? Do your shoulders feel relaxed? What about your feet and your hair? Can your feel your happiness in the tips of your fingers?

Now take a mental snapshot of this scene. You can return here whenever you need a break, whenever you need to feel refreshed and renewed. It only takes a couple of minutes. You just have to close your eyes and look at the snapshot again. It will all come flooding back to you: the sounds, smells, tastes, textures, colors; the feelings of happiness, peace, and self-confidence radiating out into each part of your body. No one can take this away from you. It's yours to keep and to draw on whenever you're in need.

3

Am I at Risk?:
Biological, Psychological,
and Relationship Risk Factors

Your Risk Profile

If you're going through the pain of a postpartum reaction, you've probably asked yourself many times, "Why me?" After all, you took good care
of yourself during your pregnancy; you have a beautiful baby and a loving husband—this should be the happiest time of your life. The problem
is, it's not. So where did you go wrong? The answer is that you didn't.

The causes of postpartum reactions are varied and complex. For the
purposes of helping you sort out your own risk profile, we've organized
these causes into three general categories: biological, psychological, and
what we're calling relationship causes. You're likely to find some combination of these factors at the root of your postpartum reaction. This chapter includes a questionnaire that may help you see the pattern of cause
and effect in your own particular situation. We've explained each risk
factor in some detail, providing case histories along the way.

As you begin to consider some of the factors that may have contributed to what you're going through, be gentle with yourself. Don't use
this information to blame or criticize yourself—you've probably done
enough of that already. Instead, set the blaming aside, put on your prob-
lem-solving cap, and see if you can find and fit together the matching
puzzle pieces. By identifying some of the influences that caused your
postpartum reaction, you'll come closer to being able to change your en-
vironmental support system, and circumstances, in ways that will ultimately make you feel better.

The Postpartum Risk Profile Questionnaire

Even though you may not be an expert on postpartum adjustment, you are an expert on yourself and your postpartum experience. As you fill out the risk profile questionnaire, keep an open mind about what may be causing your difficulties, and think about how well each possible reason fits or doesn't fit for you. The questionnaire will help you organize your responses and ideas. We've provided a sample of a completed risk profile questionnaire to give you a clearer picture of the depth and detail of responses we have in mind.

Your Risk Profile Questionnaire

For each item, circle how much you think this risk factor has affected you, contributing to your postpartum problems. Use the blank lines following each section to add any relevant information that wasn't covered. Refer to the explanations of each risk factor in the text that follows this questionnaire.

Biological Factors   **How much has this factor affected you? (Circle the best response.)**

1. Normal physical changes of   not at all   a little   a lot
pregnancy and childbirth
Comments: _____

_____

2. Hormonal changes of pregnancy   not at all   a little   a lot
and childbirth
Comments: _____

_____

3. Heredity   not at all   a little   a lot
Comments: _____

_____

4. A previous episode of postpartum   not at all   a little   a lot
reaction
Comments: _____

_____

5. Complications of pregnancy and   not at all   a little   a lot
childbirth
Comments: _____

_____

6. Breastfeeding and weaning   not at all   a little   a lot
Comments: _____

_____

7. PMS and other menstrual problems   not at all   a little   a lot
Comments: _____

_____

Your Risk Profile Questionnarie (continued)

8. Thyroid imbalance   not at all   a little   a lot
Comments: _____

_____

Other biological factors not mentioned: _____

_____

_____

_____

Psychological Factors   **How much has this factor affected you? (Circle the best response.)**

9. Normal psychological changes   not at all   a little   a lot
accompanying childbirth
Comments: _____

10. Expectations about motherhood   not at all   a little a lot
Comments: _____

11. Lifestyle patterns   not at all   a little   a lot
Comments: _____

12. Previous   not at all   a little   a lot
psychological problems
Comments: _____

13. Childhood   not at all   a little   a lot
experiences
Comments: _____

14. Unresolved losses   not at all   a little   a lot
Comments: _____

15. Recent stressful life events   not at all   a little   a lot
Comments: _____

16. Personal resources for self-care   not at all   a little   a lot
and coping
Comments: _____

Other psychological factors not mentioned: _____

_____

_____

_____

Your Risk Profile Questionnarie (continued)

Relationship Factors	How much has this factor affected you? (Circle the best response.)		
17. Normal relationship changes following childbirth	not at all	a little	a lot
Comments: _____			
18. The quality of your marriage or partnership	not at all	a little	a lot
Comments: _____			
19. The quality of your social support system	not at all	a little	a lot
Comments: _____			
20. Being a single mom	not at all	a little	a lot
Comments: _____			
21. The quality of your relationship with your baby	not at all	a little	a lot
Comments: _____			
22. Your relationship with your other children	not at all	a little	a lot
Comments: _____			

Other relationship factors not mentioned: _____
_____
_____
_____

Once you've constructed a plausible picture of what led to your postpartum problems, share the results with your partner, a therapist, or a trusted friend. It can be difficult to see yourself clearly, especially when you are going through so many changes at once. Getting an outside perspective can provide valuable information. Remind yourself again to use this information as an opportunity to learn something new, but not as an occasion for judgment. After you're done with your assessment, put your risk profile questionnaire away for a few days, and then take it out again. Time is also a valuable source of perspective. Decide if there's anything you want to add or change. You can fill out the questionnaire first, or you can read this chapter first—whichever way feels most comfortable to you.

Sample Risk Profile Questionaire

For each item, circle how much you think this risk factor has affected you, contributing to your postpartum problems. Use the blank lines following each section to add any relevant information that wasn't covered. Refer to the explanations of each risk factor in the text that follows this questionnaire.

Biological Factors   **How much has this factor affected you? (Circle the best response.)**

1. Normal physical changes of preg-   not at all   (*a little*)   a lot
nancy and childbirth

Comments: I feel more tired and have less energy than I used to. I used to be so active. I don't like this change.

2. Hormonal changes of pregnancy   not at all   (*a little*)   a lot
and childbirth

Comments: _____

3. Heredity   not at all   a little   (*a lot*)

Comments: My mom had postpartum problems after my birth. So did my sister with her second child.

4. A previous episode of postpartum   (*not at all*)   a little   a lot
reaction

Comments: _____

5. Complications of   not at all   (*a little*)   a lot
pregnancy and childbirth

Comments: I had a long and difficult labor.

6. Breastfeeding and weaning   not at all   a little   (*a lot*)

Comments: I wanted to breastfeed but I didn't have enough milk. I feel really bad about this.

7. PMS and other   (*not at all*)   a little   a lot
menstrual problems

Comments: _____

8. Thyroid imbalance   (*not at all*)   a little   a lot

Comments: _____

Other biological factors not mentioned: _____

_____

_____

_____

Psychological Factors   **How much has this factor affected you? (Circle the best response.)**

9. Normal psychological changes   not at all   a little   (*a lot*)
accompanying childbirth

Comments: I don't feel like my old self. I'm uncertain about being a mother. I want my life back the way it was.

Sample Risk Profile Questionaire (continued)

Psychological Factors   **How much has this factor affected you? (Circle the best response.)**

10. Expectations about motherhood   not at all   (*a little*)   a lot

Comments: I worry sometimes whether I'm a good enough mom.

11. Lifestyle patterns   not at all   a little   (*a lot*)

Comments: I waited 8 years to have this baby, until my marriage and career were in place. I thought it would make my life complete. Instead, I feel tired and disappointed.

12. Previous psychological problems   (*not at all*)   a little   a lot

Comments: _____

13. Childhood experiences   (*not at all*)   a little   a lot

Comments: _____

14. Unresolved losses   (*not at all*)   a little   a lot

Comments: _____

15. Recent stressful life events   not at all   (*a little*)   a lot

Comments: I changed jobs about a year ago. I'm uncertain how my boss feels about my maternity leave.

16. Personal resources for self-care and coping   (*not at all*)   a little   a lot

Comments: _____

Other psychological factors not mentioned: _____

_____

_____

_____

Relationship Factors   **How much has this factor affected you? (Circle the best response.)**

17. Normal relationship changes following childbirth   not at all   (*a little*)   a lot

Comments: I miss spending time with my husband. Becoming parents has challenged our relationship.

18. The quality of your marriage or partnership   (*not at all*)   a little   a lot

Comments: _____

19. The quality of your social support system   not at all   (*a little*)   a lot

Comments: I don't want to ask my friends for help. I feel like I should be able to do this on my own.

Sample Risk Profile Questionaire (continued)

20. Being a single mom   (not at all)   a little   a lot

Comments: _____

21. The quality of your relationship   (not at all)   a little   a lot
with your baby

Comments: _____

22. Your relationship with your other   (not at all)   a little   a lot
children

Comments: _____

Other relationship factors not mentioned: _____

_____

_____

_____

Scoring Your Risk Profile Questionnaire

Once you have completed your risk profile questionnaire, score 0 points for each response of "not at all," 1 point for each response of "a little," and 2 points for each response of "a lot." If your total score equals 0-14 points, you are likely to have only mild postpartum problems. Follow the recommendations in Chapter 4. If you don't feel better within two to four weeks, seek a professional evaluation.

If your total score equals 0-14 points, *but* you had at least four two-point responses, you may want to seek a professional evaluation now.

If your total score equals 15-29 points, you are likely to have moderate postpartum problems. Reread Chapter 2 to see if your difficulties fit one of these categories. If so, read Chapter 7 to determine what kinds of additional help you may need. You can also follow the recommendations in Chapter 4, and see what effect this has. *But* if you do not feel better within one to two weeks, seek professional help using the guidelines in Chapter 7.

If your total score equals 30-44 points, you are likely to have severe postpartum problems. Seek professional help immediately. *Chances are you will need this to get better.* Read Chapter 7 to decide what to do. Follow the suggestions in Chapter 4 to aid your recovery, *but* do not use this in place of professional help.

One word of caution in scoring your questionnaire. Clinically, it has been shown that some categories of responses put you more "at risk" for a postpartum reaction than others. For example, having a previous postpartum reaction may increase your odds of having another one up to 50 percent. Read in this chapter about each item for which you scored "a lot." If you scored "a lot" for two or three items that increase your odds of having a postpartum reaction, you may be having severe problems, despite an otherwise low score.

Whatever your score, seek professional help if your problems are causing you serious concern or are crippling your ability to function in your daily life.

Biological Causes

Biology is the first category of causes that contribute to postpartum reactions. Biological causes include:

- Normal physical changes of pregnancy and childbirth
- Hormonal changes of pregnancy and childbirth
- Heredity
- A previous episode of postpartum reaction
- Complications of pregnancy and childbirth
- Breastfeeding and weaning
- Premenstrual syndrome (PMS) and other menstrual problems
- Thyroid imbalance

Each of these factors is covered separately on the risk profile questionnaire. As you fill out your questionnaire, "not at all," "a little," or "a lot," depending on how much you think a particular factor relates to you and your personal history, you may want to add comments or explanations in the space provided, especially if you circled "a lot" for a particular item. Add any additional information in the blank lines at the end of each section. Trust yourself, and your knowledge of your body, to determine which biological influences are affecting you the most.

1. Normal Physical Changes of Pregnancy and Childbirth

From the moment of conception, your body is hard at work to support you and the new life growing inside of you. The production of estrogen and progesterone increases enormously, bringing about miraculous and massive changes. Your uterus expands from the size of a small pear to the size of a football, and the skin over your belly stretches as your abdomen grows. Your chest widens so that you can take in enough air for both you and your baby. Your breasts become swollen and heavy to prepare for lactation. The amount of blood that circulates in your body is doubled, and your heart, liver, and kidneys must work that much harder to support the two of you. Long before you can feel your baby move, you will be assaulted by a host of both internal and external changes.

Different women have different physical reactions to the surge of hormones during pregnancy. You may have felt great or you may have felt sick for the entire nine months. Some women have no morning sickness at all, while others feel nauseated 24 hours a day. You may have had any number of pregnancy symptoms, from heartburn to backaches (especially during the last three months). At the end of 40 weeks, your body will be dramatically different than it was at the start of your pregnancy, and then it will be time for everything to change again.

The changes that accompany labor and delivery are as massive as the changes brought about by pregnancy—but they happen much faster. From the moment of your baby's birth, your body takes a nosedive from a pregnant to a nonpregnant state. Following childbirth, you lose much of the extra fluid you gained during pregnancy. You may experience cramping, as your uterus contracts; your bottom may be sore for a few days to several weeks, particularly if you had to have stitches to repair a tear or an episiotomy. Hemorrhoids, constipation, and difficulty urinating are all common postpartum reactions. Your breasts may become engorged with milk, feeling hard and painful. As your hormones plummet, you may feel blue or weepy for no reason at all.

With only 12-48 hours' rest in the hospital, you've barely recovered from the physical exhaustion of labor and delivery when you are sent home. Then the nighttime feedings begin, and overwhelming fatigue unlike anything you have ever known. Just getting up from a chair can become a challenge. You may feel 80 years old. If you are breastfeeding, your baby nursing can seem to occupy most of your time. Whether breastfeeding or bottle-feeding, you may wonder how in the world you can take care of your new baby while you feel so exhausted and drained. One new mom told us, "I thought after labor and delivery I was home free. I had no idea of what was ahead of me." Given the tremendous physical demands of pregnancy, childbirth, and having a new baby, it's amazing that more women do not respond with severe postpartum reactions. Treat yourself with care as you adjust to these physical changes, bearing in mind that your physical well-being is critical to your postpartum recovery.

2. Hormonal Changes of Pregnancy and Childbirth

Your body undergoes tremendous hormonal changes from the moment you become pregnant. Progesterone and estrogen are produced at much higher levels than normal to support the development of your baby. According to Gillian Ford, author of *What's Wrong with My Hormones*, by the second trimester of pregnancy the placenta produces 30 to 50 times the amount of progesterone and estrogen your body usually makes. To prepare you for nursing, prolactin levels rise. Other hormones are suddenly produced in abundance, including adrenal hormone and human chorionic gonadotropin (HCG), which is produced only during pregnancy. These hormones make possible the physical changes necessary to sustain you and your growing baby. With this increase in hormonal activity, many women report feeling better than ever. In fact, it appears that some of these hormones, progesterone in particular, may act on the brain in ways that diminish depression in much the same way as antidepressant medications.

After your baby and the placenta are delivered, your levels of estrogen and progesterone take a nosedive. Progesterone falls to zero within one week and estrogen diminishes to about 1/200th of its level during pregnancy. Four other hormones unique to pregnancy disappear altogether. At the same time, prolactin, the hormone that signals your breasts to make the changes needed for lactation, inhibits your body's production of progesterone and estrogen, especially if you breastfeed your baby. According to Katherina Dalton, author of *Depression After Childbirth*, your prolactin levels may remain high for as long as two months even if you do not breastfeed. So, whether you nurse or not, it may take a while for normal progesterone and estrogen production to resume.

What this means is that within a very short time from your child's birth, your body goes through a massive withdrawal from the hormones it became so accustomed to during pregnancy. This is just another part of the tremendous physical upheaval you are experiencing. Changes in your hormones, which are chemicals normally produced by your body, can result in significant changes in your mood and behavior. If you don't feel as chipper as you did in your second trimester, when your hormones were surging, this is completely normal. It will take time for your body to find its balance again. In response to these hormonal changes, about 80 percent of all women who give birth will experience an episode of the baby blues. You may feel weepy, sad, irritable, or moody. By the end of six to eight weeks after delivery, these completely normal feelings usually subside.

Important Note

If you're concerned that changes in your mood and behavior have become too extreme or lasted too long, you should consult your obstetrician, nurse midwife, or another health-care practitioner. If you have extreme symptoms—such as insomnia or thoughts about harming yourself or your baby—you should get in immediate touch with your health-care provider. If your symptoms persist beyond one month postpartum, arrange for a physical and psychological evaluation. Your doctor may recommend hormonal testing if this hasn't been done already, or evaluation by a health-care provider who specializes in postpartum problems. Don't assume that your symptoms will go away on their own. Especially if they are left untreated, they may get much worse. Be aggressive about getting whatever treatment and support you may need. Turn to Chapter 7 for an overview of the kinds of help available for particular problems and symptoms.

3. Heredity

Heredity describes how a particular characteristic is inherited through the genes passed on to you from your parents and the family gene pool. The difficulty in looking at this risk for postpartum adjustment problems factor is that it's impossible to know to what extent you may have biologically inherited a certain characteristic from your parents, as opposed to having psychologically acquired it through the experiences you had growing up in your family. Scholars refer to this as the "nature versus nurture" issue. With postpartum reactions, some experts think that biological inheritance has no relevance, or has at most a very weak influence. Other equally credible experts think that both biological and psychological inheritance contribute substantially to postpartum reactions and need to be considered in detail. We lean toward the latter point of view, that heredity appears to be a risk factor for postpartum reactions.

If you have a history of bi-polar or manic-depressive illness in your family, you may be especially prone to postpartum reactions. You may also be more susceptible if your mom had a postpartum reaction. The more positively you respond to the following four questions, the more likely it is that heredity has a part in your postpartum difficulties. Give a yes or no answer to the questions below:

1. Did my mom, grandmother, sisters, or other close female relatives experience a postpartum reaction?

2. Is there any history of bi-polar or manic-depressive illness in my family, including my mom, dad, siblings, grandparents, or other close relatives?

3. Is there any history of depression or anxiety in my family, including my mom, dad, siblings, grandparents, or other close relatives?

4. Have my mom, grandmother, sisters, or other close female relatives experienced any hormone-related problems, including PMS or problems at menopause?

If you don't know the answers to these questions, speak with your mom or someone else in the family who may have this information. Talk to several family members if needed, to get as complete a picture as possible. You may learn things about your family you didn't know before. Other female relatives may be relieved to finally share their postpartum experiences with someone who understands. By speaking with your family, you may feel less alone and less "different." Whatever happens, congratulate yourself on bringing up these questions with your family, and looking for answers.

4. A Previous Episode of Postpartum Reaction

One thing that the experts do agree on is that if you've experienced one postpartum reaction, you're more likely to have another one. Some studies suggest that the chances of this happening to you again are as high as 50 percent. If these odds alarm you, keep in mind that most women do not get medical or psychological help for their postpartum problems. With treatment, these odds may be a lot lower. Anyway, the sooner you get help, the speedier your recovery will be. If you are going through a postpartum reaction, be certain to seek whatever help you need until you are symptom-free and feel like your old self again—or as much like your old self as possible within the context of having a brand-new baby. A full physical and emotional recovery from your present postpartum problems is the best insurance against a future postpartum reaction. Specific guidelines for determining the kinds of help you may need are presented in Chapter 7.

If you have been through a previous postpartum reaction, and are pregnant or thinking about getting pregnant, start designing a plan for good prenatal and postpartum care now. Don't wait until your baby is born. Early intervention is the best way to prevent another postpartum reaction. Get all the help you need, and be sure to discuss your previous postpartum difficulties with your health-care team. We talk more about what you can do to prevent the recurrence of a postpartum reaction in Chapter 9, "Before the Storm."

Lisa had her first postpartum reaction when she was 28. Within days following her daughter's birth, she slipped into a manic episode— she felt boundless energy, but got little done, sleeping only a few hours a night regardless of the baby's schedule. Her husband and friends noticed that she seemed to be speaking faster than she could think. As the days passed, Lisa's mania gave way to depression: she felt hopeless and disappointed in herself. She felt that her problems were her own fault, and reasoned that she must be a horrible person to be feeling this way.

When she became pregnant with her second child, Lisa spoke to her OB, who referred her to a psychiatrist who specialized in postpartum reactions. "I knew I couldn't go through another birth like that. I thought I'd rather die. I didn't know what was happening to me, and I didn't know how to stop it."

The psychiatrist sent her to a psychologist who worked with postpartum moms. In therapy, Lisa learned about the causes of postpartum depression, what most likely triggered her problems, and what she could do differently this time. She had a chance to work through her feelings and concerns that resulted from her first postpartum reaction, and to grieve her suffering and shattered expectations. Her new health-care team followed her closely throughout her pregnancy and following the birth of her second daughter. When Lisa began to exhibit some manic symptoms a few days after her baby's delivery, Lisa quickly got the medical care and psychological support she needed. Her symptoms did not get out of hand, and she had the chance "to be the kind of mom I always wanted to be from the start."

5. Complications of Pregnancy and Childbirth

Like heredity, the extent to which problems during pregnancy and childbirth contribute to postpartum difficulties is difficult to pin down. Still, most women would agree that the conditions of pregnancy and the nature of their birth experience have a profound effect on them later on. Maybe you were confined to bed rest for the last ten weeks of your pregnancy because of bleeding, or went into premature labor and had to be hospitalized, in terror that your baby would be born too soon to survive. Maybe you planned to have a vaginal birth and ended up with a C-section instead, or planned to deliver without any pain medication and changed your mind. Maybe your husband was absent when you went into labor, or your own OB didn't make it to the delivery. While some of these situations might be considered typical complications, they are still ways in which your pregnancy and delivery may have differed from what you expected. Because of this, the memory of these complications may be contributing to your postpartum problems.

Every woman has her own set of ideas and hopes about what her pregnancy and birth experience will be like. To the extent that yours was different from what you expected, you may be more likely to have a postpartum reaction. If you had a C-section or another emergency procedure or hospitalization, you may be feeling depressed about being cheated of a "normal" childbirth experience. If you developed complications after your delivery, or your baby required special medical care, you may have suffered a good deal of anxiety and fear. Sometimes when complications arise, the extra support you received from family and friends will head off postpartum difficulties. But sometimes there's not an adequate support system in place, or the complications are just too traumatic for any amount of support to help.

Take time now to reflect on the circumstances of your pregnancy and childbirth experience. Ask yourself how they compared with what you hoped for. Be aware of your feelings as you remember, and think about how they may be adding to your current distress.

6. Breastfeeding and Weaning

From a biological standpoint, the hormonal changes related to breastfeeding and weaning may put you more at risk for a postpartum reaction. While you are nursing, prolactin levels remain high. This interferes with your body's production of estrogen and progesterone to restore your already depleted supply of these hormones. When you stop nursing, it may take a while for your prolactin levels to fall, and your body's normal production of estrogen and progesterone to resume. In addition, weaning may lead to a drop in your endorphin levels because of lowered prolactin production. Endorphins are naturally occurring body chemicals that give people a sense of well-being—so you might not feel too well when you wean, especially if you wean suddenly.

Besides hormonal changes, nursing is a physically demanding activity, and you may soon feel that it's all you ever do. If you are nursing you may have less freedom to be away from your baby, and to care for yourself than you would if your baby was bottle-fed. You may feel as if your baby is permanently attached to your bosom. You may feel like a contortionist as you learn to do everything—from going to the bathroom to putting on your shoes—while supporting a nursing baby in the crook of your arm.

Given the hormonal changes in your body, and the amount of time and energy you expend on nursing, it would seem that weaning should put you less at risk for a postpartum reaction. But, for most women, this isn't the case. How can this be explained? For many moms, nursing is a time of special closeness with their babies, and weaning signals the end of this time. If you were happy with your nursing experience, you may be sad that this time of special closeness has ended. If you had to stop nursing before you were ready because of physical problems—because someone said that your baby wasn't getting enough milk, or you had to stop so that you could take medications—your grief may be especially strong. You may be telling yourself that you're a failure because this happened; that this is further proof of your inadequacy as a mom. This kind of negative "self-talk" often leads to depression, and may be part of your present difficulties.

If you've been nursing your baby for a long time, giving this up may be an even greater loss for you. The more important nursing has been to you, the stronger your feelings about weaning are bound to be. Remember this in thinking about how the process of weaning is affecting you now. Think about what nursing has meant to you, and what your expectations were. As in the case of pregnancy and childbirth, it's not necessarily what has happened, but what you tell yourself about what's happened, that may be contributing to your problems. If you are saying such things to yourself as, "I had problems nursing, so I've failed as a mom," or "I will never feel this close to my child again," you are likely to feel sad and upset. How you feel depends on what your experience of nursing has been, what you say to yourself about it, and any related feelings of grieving or loss you may have.

7. PMS and Other Menstrual Problems

In both premenstrual syndrome (PMS) and postpartum reactions, many symptoms can be attributed to hormones. Changes in both mood and behavior can result from changes in the levels of progesterone, estrogen, and other reproductive hormones produced by your body. During your monthly cycle, estrogen and progesterone—as well as other significant reproductive hormones—are at their lowest levels just before your period starts. Typically, women report the most premenstrual symptoms in the first few days before their periods begin, and during the first few days of their period, when the levels of these hormones are at their lowest ebb. For some women, symptoms will occur at other times during the two weeks prior to menstruation.

Now, consider how dramatically your hormones plummet following childbirth. For women who already suffer from PMS, such changes can rapidly result in a postpartum reaction. But the connection between PMS and postpartum reactions is much more complicated. For reasons that are not fully understood, clinical accounts suggest that once a woman experiences a postpartum reaction, her chance of experiencing PMS also rises, even if she never had any prior premenstrual symptoms. Katherina Dalton, a pioneer in PMS and postpartum problems, has concluded that a woman with no history of PMS has a 90 percent chance of developing it after she experiences a postpartum reaction.

If you are currently having postpartum difficulties, you may find that your symptoms get worse sometime in the premenstrual phase of your cycle. Remember, this worsening of symptoms occurs at different times in the menstrual cycle, depending on the individual woman involved. You may notice that you feel the worst a few days or two weeks before your period, anywhere to several days after your period. You may also have some months in which you don't experience many symptoms at all.

Monitor when your PMS occurs, so that you can plan for it. Try to leave more stressful tasks for other times of the month. Do what you can throughout the month to follow a healthy diet, take vitamin and mineral supplements as needed, exercise two to three times a week, and get proper rest. Your PMS may not go away, but you can learn to manage it better. To read more about PMS and what you can do, consult *Unmasking PMS,* by Joseph Martorano, M.D., and Maureen Morgan, C.S.W., R.N.

8. Thyroid Imbalance

Following childbirth, the level of hormones produced by your thyroid drops lower than it was before you were pregnant. Like progesterone and estrogen, thyroid hormones carry messages to your brain that regulate internal body functions, including temperature control and energy level. When the production of these hormones is low, you may feel exhausted, slowed down, and sluggish. You may also experience weight gain, dry skin, constipation, and heavier than normal periods when your periods resume. Other symptoms of low thyroid may include mood swings, severe agitation, fatigue, trouble sleeping, and tension. If your production of these hormones is too high, you may feel overanxious and speeded up. Clearly, the under- or over-production of thyroid results in physical changes that can affect your emotional well-being.

The decrease in thyroid functioning that may follow childbirth is further aggravated by an increased production of the hormone prolactin. As we said earlier, prolactin increases to prepare your body for nursing; but this increase can cause either a temporary or permanent condition of low thyroid after pregnancy. Even for women who do not nurse, prolactin levels may remain elevated for several months postpartum. If you are nursing, prolactin will remain elevated until you stop. Although problems in thyroid functioning are relatively rare postpartum, you might want to have your thyroid measured if you're experiencing weight gain and feelings of sluggishness.

Thyroid problems can develop from other hormonal changes after childbirth. Because the various hormone systems in your body are intimately connected, and influence each other, there are many potential breakdowns in the system following a significant reproductive event like childbirth. This is why women with a postpartum reaction, PMS, or menopausal difficulties may have multiple hormonal imbalances, including progesterone or estrogen deficiencies, excess prolactin, and/or thyroid dysfunction. Often, it's difficult to isolate one particular source for a set of such problems. Instead, there may be many different circuits misfiring from your brain, to your glands (thyroid, pituitary, ovaries, adrenals), to your cells.

If you feel overly sluggish or have had significant postpartum weight gain, consult your doctor for possible thyroid involvement. He or she may want to evaluate you, and may possibly refer you to a specialist for additional testing. If there is any history of thyroid problems in your family, be certain to report this.

Thyroid imbalance can be a complicated problem to sort out. Have patience, but persist until you are satisfied with the outcome. If your postpartum difficulties are the result of thyroid dysfunction, or are being intensified by it, you'll need appropriate medical intervention before you can feel better.

Psychological Causes

Psychology is the second main category of factors that can contribute to postpartum reactions. Psychological risk factors include:

- Normal psychological changes accompanying childbirth
- Expectations about motherhood
- Lifestyle patterns
- Previous psychological problems
- Childhood experiences
- Unresolved losses
- Recent stressful life events
- Personal resources for self-care and coping

Each of these categories is an item on the risk profile questionnaire.

9. Normal Psychological Changes Accompanying Childbirth

Even as your body is assaulted by the physical upheaval of childbirth, you are faced with tremendous psychological changes. Having a baby changes the way you see yourself and look at your life, forever. So, why doesn't anyone mention this when they're wheeling you out of the hospital with your new son or daughter in your arms? The most likely reason is "the motherhood myth." For some odd and outdated reason, becoming a mom is still not fully regarded as a time of enormous biological, psychological, emotional, and interpersonal change. Instead, the idea persists that once you physically give birth, you became a mom psychologically and emotionally, too. The truth is that giving birth is only the first small step in your journey to motherhood.

Probably the biggest psychological challenge you will face is figuring out who you are now that you have a baby, and what motherhood is about for you. At first, being a mom may be most tied to meeting your baby's physical demands. Caring for a newborn can be so physically and emotionally consuming that who you are seems to get lost in the shuffle. Whether you worked outside your home before your pregnancy or not, you may quickly forget that you ever did anything besides change dirty diapers and wipe spit-up from your baby's face. Although extremely important, these kinds of activities do not tend to increase your self-esteem or offer a new view of yourself that's particularly appealing.

Elizabeth, a 39-year-old TV reporter who had waited eight years to have children, told us: "I couldn't believe when I brought my new son home that this was what I had waited for all these years. I told myself that becoming a mom would make my life complete, and enhance my sense of myself. Overnight, I went from being a successful TV journalist to a wet nurse. I felt cheated and misled." If your old sense of yourself has been temporarily shattered, this is normal. Slowly but surely, you will begin to put the pieces back together again. The hope is that becoming a mom will enlarge your sense of yourself, as Lyn Delliquadri and Kati

Breckenridge suggest in their book *Mother Care*. But, for now, you may feel that you've lost both your old self and your sense of self-worth, and have little idea about what lies ahead.

If you feel like your world has been turned upside down, it has. Before your baby was born, you probably spent most of your time doing what you chose, whether work or leisure activities. Not that you always liked what you did; but most likely you set your own schedule and were free to come and go as you pleased. This is a second psychological challenge you'll encounter. Since your baby has arrived, you must decide how to combine motherhood with the rest of your life. As you explore your current thoughts and feelings, set aside any ideas you had during your pregnancy about how this would work. Many women have preconceived ideas about motherhood, and run into trouble when things don't work out the way they'd planned.

Nancy, a 28-year-old RN, told us that she'd planned to stay home full-time after having her baby, "but I was losing my mind! The more I pushed myself to make it work, the worse I got. Finally, I became so depressed I couldn't get out of bed in the morning. With my husband's and family's support, I went back to work, and started to feel better after a couple of weeks."

Remember, you have the right to decide and re-decide what will work out best for you. The decision you make may vary at different points in your life, and with different pregnancies. Make time for yourself, whether you work inside or outside of your home, to do the things you enjoyed before your baby came. You may not have as much time, but you can still find *some* time to take care of yourself.

As your baby grows and changes, your sense of who you are and your role as a mother is also likely to change. Over time, physical demands will diminish, and emotional rewards will increase. The first time your baby smiles at you, you will feel renewed by this gift of love and affection. You may also feel scared as you realize the great responsibility you have undertaken. With each milestone your child reaches, new feelings may be kindled inside of you about what motherhood means. Keep in mind always that becoming a mom does not happen overnight, or on the first day you bring your baby home. It's a lifelong process that is constantly changing and unfolding. Be patient with yourself. You have plenty of time.

10. Expectations of Motherhood

Even before you became pregnant, you probably thought about what you would be like as a mom, and how you would approach motherhood. Typically, these expectations are based on what you experienced with your own mom, on culturally shared attitudes about motherhood, and on your ideas about what "good" mothers are like. The problem is that you may have set your expectations too high, and are angry with yourself now for falling so short of them.

If you expect yourself to always know what to do, and to do the right thing all the time, you're likely to feel both disappointed and distressed. Being a mother is an imperfect science. It's a process of trial and error, and making many mistakes. The more perfect you expect yourself to be, the more you may find yourself buried in self-criticism and blame.

Lucy was a 34-year-old attorney who developed anxiety symptoms about six weeks after the birth of her third child. During her pregnancy, she had planned every detail of how she would spend her maternity leave. Unfortunately, her plans crumbled when she had to dismiss her children's sitter, and several other unexpected problems occurred. "I felt myself falling apart because I wasn't getting around to doing the things I had planned. Even though I knew it didn't make sense, I kept criticizing myself for not sticking to my list. I was angry and sad that my maternity leave wasn't turning out the way I expected it to, and I couldn't stop blaming myself for it."

Some women fall into the trap of expecting themselves to do everything in the same way they were used to doing it before their baby arrived. This may mean keeping your home spotless, or fixing a three-course dinner most nights. It may involve your determination to return to work after six weeks' leave, no matter how you feel. Perhaps you expect yourself to listen to your friends' problems whenever they need a sympathetic ear; or maybe you're accustomed to leading a fast-paced life, always on the go. If you expect your life to remain basically unchanged after you become a mother, your expectations are bound to be shattered. Remember, having a baby creates enormous physical, psychological, and interpersonal changes. Expect things to be different. Be flexible in adapting yourself to the many challenges of being a parent. The more you expect things to remain the same, the more likely you are to experience feelings of depression, anxiety, and loss.

11. Lifestyle Patterns

First-Time Moms

Becoming a mom for the first time can place you at greater risk for a postpartum reaction than women who are having their second or third child. Your life changes dramatically with the transition to parenthood; and this can't help but have a profound effect on you emotionally. As a first-time mom, you may experience strong feelings of sadness and discomfort at the loss of your old self and pre-baby lifestyle. Although childbirth is usually thought of as a time of new beginnings, it is also a time of significant losses: the loss of your pregnancy, the loss of the freedoms of being childless, the loss of being a couple as you knew it, and the loss of who you were before motherhood.

Theresa, a 37-year-old first-time mom, confided: "Before my daughter's birth, I was constantly going, and thought of myself as a very strong person. Then I had her, and little stresses which never bothered me before would reduce me to tears. I felt like I didn't know myself anymore, and what my abilities and limitations were. It was really scary. At least when my father died, I expected to feel bad for a long time, until I finished grieving. I didn't know that having a baby would be such a loss of myself, and wondered when it would end. I wish someone had told me."

If you are a first-time mom, your expectations of yourself may be too high for several reasons. If you have no direct experience with motherhood, you may have drawn your images of what it would be like from TV commercials and magazine ads showing beautiful, calm, rested moms with their cheerful, angelic babies. You may think that you should be like this too—always smiling, content, and patient. Think again. This picture is about as far from the reality of new motherhood as you can get; but you may continue to feel let down that your experience is so different. To make up for the difference, you may push yourself to be a more "perfect" mom—and the more you do, the more difficulties you're likely to create for yourself.

Even if you anticipated some stress with becoming a new mom, it's impossible to understand in your gut the enormous changes you'll go through until you experience them. As is the case with leaving home, marriage, and other significant life changes, your idea of what these changes will be like is often very different from your actual experience of them. No matter how modest your expectations about motherhood may have been, it's likely that they were still unrealistic. If you are able to care for your baby, and take some time to care for yourself, you will be doing well. During the first six months, the physical and emotional demands of being a new mom are tremendous. If you find the time to do a load of laundry or make a nice dinner, pat yourself on the back. Expect little of yourself, and give yourself a lot of credit for what you are able to do.

One friend of ours said that she decided, when her baby was born, to forgive herself in advance for all the mistakes and wrong decisions she'd inevitably make during the course of her career as a mother. This kind of attitude can help you weather your disappointment in yourself at those times (and they'll come!) when you fall short of your ideal.

Older Moms

Today, more women are waiting longer to have children. Although delayed child-bearing offers some definite advantages, it may also put you more at risk for a postpartum reaction. This is, again, because of the inevitable upheaval in your lifestyle, and the opportunity for you to have developed unrealistically high expectations about motherhood. By the time you become a mom, you may have already spent 10-15 years working, and be well-established in your career. You've probably grown used to spending your time as you choose, and may have a fairly set routine of work and leisure activities. No matter how long you've been planning to have a baby, the reality of actually becoming a mom is likely to be more tumultuous than anything you imagined. You may be having problems adjusting to your baby's routine because of the ways in which it's interfering with your own. This is not a sign of selfishness, but rather a reaction to how much your life has changed. You may yearn for your morning cup of coffee, reading the newspaper, or working out at the gym. You may feel angry, guilty, or depressed, because you love your baby but desperately miss your old life.

As a woman of the world, you may have especially high expectations of yourself. You may think that you ought to have this all figured out by now, and you may be allowing yourself far too little margin for error. Perhaps you expect that you'll be able to handle motherhood in the same controlled and organized way in which you've managed the rest of your life. After all, how difficult can caring for a newborn be? By this time in your life, you're likely to have encountered many difficult situations, and have had success in coping with them. Certainly, this can't be that much different! But it is, and the more you expect yourself to deal with motherhood rationally, without making a lot of mistakes, the more you raise your risk for a postpartum reaction.

It may help to remember that there's no such thing as a perfect mother. Mistakes are part of the process with each child.

Perfectionism, Negative Thinking, and the Need for Control

Like first-time moms and older moms, women with certain personality characteristics seem to be more at risk for postpartum problems than women who do not have these traits. The main three personality characteristics that appear to put you at higher risk for a postpartum reaction are

- Need for control

- Perfectionism, accompanied by high expectations

- A tendency toward negative thinking and excessive worrying

The greater your need for control, the more having a baby is likely to create problems for you. For the most part, your baby's needs will dictate what you do and when, and there is little you can do to change this. Your baby will let you know when he/she needs to be fed, changed, rocked, or walked. Your baby's sleeping habits will influence yours, and if she needs a bottle at 12:30 a.m. and again at 2:30 a.m., she won't stop crying until you satisfy her. Your daily routine will undergo major revisions; the constant sense of disruption and unpredictability may leave you feeling unsettled and frustrated. No matter how organized you were before your baby was born, you're not likely to have the energy to maintain your old standards postpartum. You will feel at the mercy of your body and your hormones, as your milk leaks when your baby cries and you tear up over the Saturday night news. In many ways, you will not be in control, and you may despair over this.

Jessica, a 37-year-old professional, talked to us about how her mom warned her that her days of "being in control" would end with the birth of her first daughter. "My mom told me that I had my life wrapped up in these neat little packages, which were about to fall apart—and I didn't know how right she was. I still expected my life to be about the same. I didn't realize how accustomed I'd become to doing things 'my way.' I thought we would fit the baby into our routine except for her sleep schedule; but she had other ideas. I felt depressed about my lack of control over my life, and wondered if things would ever get better."

Being a perfectionist and having high expectations of yourself can also add to your risk of experiencing a postpartum reaction. Very often, perfectionism and a need for control exist side by side. Just as it's impossible to control the changes associated with having a new baby, being a perfect mother defies the reality of postpartum adjustment (it defies *any* reality!). The higher your expectations are, the further you have to fall. If you expect yourself to be your best when you are going through a time of enormous physical and emotional change, you are setting yourself up to fail. Over time, this sense of failure can diminish your self-esteem, and lead to postpartum problems.

We can't say it often enough—being a mom is an imperfect science, and learning to be a good mother isn't something that happens overnight. Motherhood is a process of trial and error, and everyone makes lots of mistakes along the way. Caring for a newborn is an incredibly demanding task, maybe the hardest thing you have ever done. Congratulate yourself for what you are doing. Most likely, you are doing much more than you're giving yourself credit for.

Excessive worry and negative thinking can also increase your chances of having postpartum difficulties. How you think about things influences how you feel. The more worrying and negative thinking you do, the more you may set yourself up to feel unhappy and distressed. This is especially true when you're dealing with such a major life change as having a baby. For all mothers, childbirth brings with it numerous concerns, including the immense responsibility of caring for your new baby's physical and emotional well-being. When you combine these normal worries with a habit of worrying and seeing things negatively, your chances of having a postpartum reaction increase considerably.

You may find yourself overly concerned with your baby's health, and be preoccupied with every cough and sneeze. You may see a car accident on TV, and start imagining that something similar will happen to your child. You may think about your infant as a teenager, and feel fearful and distressed about all the dangers held in store by the future.

If you're a worrier, your negative thinking may be focused on yourself, as well as your child, on how you are not doing well. You may have concerns about your physical recovery, or about getting your pre-baby figure back. You may worry that you are having emotional problems, and will never feel like yourself again. You may tell yourself that you are not being a good mother—that you are not doing anything worthwhile. The more you worry and think negatively about what you are going through, the more likely you will be to have trouble coping with postpartum changes.

12. Previous Psychological Problems

If you have already experienced one or more episodes of depression, anxiety, or psychosis in your life, you're probably at higher risk for a postpartum reaction. If your prior episode of depression, anxiety, or psychosis occurred following childbirth, your odds of this happening again are potentially one in two. You will want to check this category off on your risk profile questionnaire, whether or not you were ever diagnosed as having psychological problems, and whether or not you ever received treatment for your difficulties. Even today, many people feel ashamed of seeking psychological help, and suffer through their symptoms needlessly. With some problems, you can spend most of your lifetime feeling bad if you don't get help. Remember, the best insurance against another episode of psychological difficulty is prompt, effective treatment at the first onset of symptoms, for as long as you need the help.

Even if you don't have a history of anxiety, depression, or psychosis, you are more likely to have problems adjusting to motherhood if you had difficulty with other major life changes. This may include having a particularly rough time as a teenager, trouble leaving home, difficulty being married, or overwhelming problems figuring out what to do with your life. Again, it's normal to have some difficulty adjusting to these situations, because they are so big and create so much psychological and emotional change. Still, some people have more problems facing these challenges than other people do. If you've experienced trouble in dealing with major life changes, this does not mean that you're weak or defective, but it may place you at higher risk for postpartum difficulties. On the other hand, experts have estimated that the stress of motherhood alone may put anyone at a 15-times-higher risk for experiencing symptoms of emotional distress. In fact, as many as 70 percent of all women who experience a postpartum reaction have no prior history of psychological problems.

If you have a history of psychiatric or psychological problems, be sure to be forthcoming to your OB about this information—you may avoid agonizing weeks or months of horrible symptoms. Assemble the health-care team that can provide you with support and intervention if needed. Have the other members of your support network in place to keep your stress at the lowest level possible.

13. *Childhood Experiences*

Just as you influence your child's social and emotional development, you were influenced by how things were in your family when you were growing up. If you experienced physical abuse or sexual abuse as a child, you may be more at risk for a postpartum reaction. If you experienced emotional abuse or emotional neglect as a child, you may also be at higher risk for postpartum problems. Emotional abuse involves being ridiculed, criticized, put down, and overall being treated without respect. Emotional neglect is when your physical and emotional or social needs are not met by your parents or caretakers. Emotional abuse and neglect often occur in families in which one or both parents is alcoholic or mentally ill. Although there is no outward physical violence or sexual abuse, the effects can be equally devastating to a child's self-esteem and sense of identity. Whatever kind of abuse or neglect you may have endured, chances are that it lowered your self-esteem, made you feel less certain about who you are, and diminished your ability to build close personal relationships.

Now, imagine you already have some of these characteristics, and are faced with the responsibility of a new baby—which automatically challenges your sense of identity and self-esteem. This may lead to even more problems for you. If you suffered abuse or neglect as a child, postpartum adjustment may be more difficult, because you didn't observe or experience what it was like to be a "good enough" mom. Not knowing what to do may increase your anxiety and self-doubt—even women raised in relatively healthy homes struggle to feel competent. Added to this, you may find that having your own baby triggers memories and feelings of what your childhood was like. This can be very distressing, especially if you find yourself having thoughts or feelings about abusing your child in the ways in which you were abused.

Zia was a 35-year-old mother of two. From the ages of six to eleven, Zia had been sexually abused by her mother's brother, who lived with their family. She thought she had put this experience behind her. But with the birth of her second child, she found herself worrying about the possibility of molesting him as she had been molested. Zia felt very guilty about having these thoughts, and her guilt gave way to feelings of depression. She decided that she must be a horrible person and an unfit mom to be thinking such things; in her depression, she withdrew from caring for her son. It took several months of professional support before Zia was able to stop feeling like a criminal for having these thoughts, and allowed herself to have a warm and loving relationship with her son.

Not all women who have a history of abuse will experience thoughts about sexually or physically abusing their children. But if you have such a history, you need to deal with your feelings of hurt, rage, and helplessness. A child—especially a baby—is in a vulnerable relationship with the adults he or she looks to for care and support. It's a relationship that's easily abused. Don't wait until you have a child to work out your feelings about past imbalances and abuses. The best prevention against repeating the cycle of abuse is to get help before you decide to have a baby.

If you have thoughts about harming your child, read the sections in Chapter 2 about postpartum obsessive-compulsive reaction. You're unlikely to act on such thoughts so long as you know they are a problem. But it's a good idea to consider them as a signal, in any case, that you have some unresolved feelings that need to be worked out. Such thoughts can also lead, as they did in the case of Zia, above, to feelings of depression or other mood disorders. Women who have thoughts about harming themselves or their baby but whose judgment is clouded should seek professional help immediately. Refer to the section in Chapter 2 on postpartum thought reactions. In both the United States and England, more women kill their children in the first year following childbirth than at any other time. This cycle of abuse and neglect tends to repeat itself unless there is a conscious effort to stop it.

If you did not grow up in an extremely negative environment where you experienced abuse or neglect, but still had a difficult or ambivalent relationship with your mom, you may be more at risk for postpartum problems. By ambivalent we mean that you may have had feelings toward your mom that were sometimes very negative and sometimes very positive. Of course, most women will describe some mixed feelings toward their mothers; but the more extreme the ambivalence, the more problematic your own adjustment as a mother may be. You will probably not want to imitate how your mother parented you, but at times you may find yourself treating your child as your mother treated you. It is not that you intend to give your baby mixed messages or to be unloving, but these are the relationship patterns you learned.

As with abuse, these patterns tend to repeat themselves unless you become aware of what is going on and actively learn to relate differently to your child. If you didn't feel securely attached to your own mom, you may have trouble feeling consistently loving and caring toward your own baby. Don't give up hope. Seek guidance from your partner if he comes from a happier family background than your own. Read books. Attend parenting classes. Watch other moms with their babies, and think about what seems to work best, and what behaviors you'd like to avoid. Get professional help if needed. Remember, all mothers have some mixed feelings toward their children. Dealing with mixed feelings in a conscious and caring way is difficult for most parents to learn, especially if you didn't experience this kind of sensitivity from your parents. Be patient, conscientious, and persistent as you learn to relate differently to your baby. Even women who were fortunate enough to have close relationships with their moms have a lot to learn when they become parents themselves.

14. Unresolved Losses

Because having a baby is both a time of loss and a time of new beginnings, unresolved feelings about past losses may resurface. If you have not dealt with previous losses in your life, you may be more at risk for a postpartum reaction. Your unfinished business may be over the loss of a parent, spouse, or some other important person in your life. You may not have finished grieving the loss of other children, and other pregnancies. If you have experienced miscarriage, stillbirth, an ectopic pregnancy, or terminated a pregnancy, this may add to your risk. Sometimes, having a previous postpartum reaction, and not mourning the lost hopes and expectations of that childbirth experience, may intensify feelings of sadness and despair.

Your loss may involve moving to another state or city and leaving behind your family, your friends, and your sense of security. If it's a recent move, you may not have had time to mourn these changes. Even if it has been several years, your grieving may not be completed. The more significant the loss, the longer it may take you to feel emotionally settled.

Other losses may involve a job change, a friend's moving away, or health problems. Keep in mind that it is not necessarily a problem that these changes have occurred in your life. The difficulty comes when you have not dealt with your feelings about these losses, or gone through the grieving process. Despite all your best efforts, if you have not faced your feelings over past losses, they may reemerge at other turning points in your life.

15. Recent Stressful Life Events

Without any doubt, the greater the number of stressful life events you experience during pregnancy and in the immediate postpartum period, the more likely you are to have a postpartum reaction. Because pregnancy and giving birth are considered to be stressful life events on their own, the addition of other major life changes can easily tip the scales. Examples of such events include the death of someone close to you, a geographic move, a loss or change of job for you or your partner, a change in financial status, or the serious illness of someone close to you. Ironically, couples often bring about major life changes inspired by the impending birth of their child: many expectant parents suddenly decide to change careers, go back to school, remodel their house, or move. Whether an event was something you chose, or something completely out of your control, the closer it occurs to the time of your child's birth (either pre- or postpartum) the more it will add to the stresses you are already coping with. Try not to make major life changes, such as buying a new house, close to the time of your child's birth. Conserve your emotional resources for the tremendous demands of having a new baby.

Instead of making your life more demanding, do what you can to reduce current stressors. If you tend to lead your life in a stressful way, pressuring yourself with high expectations and a hectic schedule, do what you can to modify these habits. Learn relaxation techniques that will help you cope well with stressful life events when they occur. Although you can't stop life changes from happening, you may be better able to cope with them if you have a less stressful lifestyle.

16. Personal Resources for Self-Care and Coping

Researchers have found that certain emotional traits seem to decrease the risk of experiencing a postpartum reaction. One of these is your ability to cope and adjust to changes in your life—in other words, your emotional flexibility. The other is your ability to take care of yourself. Although having a baby is stressful for any woman, some women seem to have the emotional resources to cope better than others. The resources that seem to help the most are flexibility, open-mindedness, and a positive self-regard. Seeing change as an opportunity to grow as a person, and being open to new experiences, may help you cope. Being patient with yourself, and self-accepting rather than self-critical, can go a long way. The more positive, open-minded, and self-affirming you are, the less difficult your adjustment is likely to be.

Taking good care of yourself emotionally is equally important. Like the varying ability to cope with changes, it appears that some women are better at taking care of themselves than others. Taking care of yourself means making your emotional needs a priority, and taking time out to see that these needs are satisfied. It means that you see yourself as an important person in your life—as important as your partner or family or friends—and you're not afraid to say so. You know how to assert yourself with others so that they respect your needs and treat you as someone who counts. Women who take care of themselves tend to be open with their thoughts and feelings, and direct in their communications. Because of this foundation, they are more likely to apply these skills during their postpartum adjustment. This tends to enhance their emotional well-being and diminish their chances of a postpartum reaction.

Relationship Factors

Relationship factors are the third general category of influences that contribute to your risk for a postpartum reaction. These factors include:

- Normal relationship changes following childbirth
- The quality of your marriage or partnership
- The quality of your social support system
- Being a single mom
- The quality of your relationship with your baby
- Your relationship with your other children

Each of these influences appears as an item on your risk profile
questionnaire.

17. Normal Relationship Changes Following Childbirth

Just as having a baby results in tremendous physical and psychological changes, it also brings about significant relationship changes. If
you didn't hear about this in your Lamaze class, don't be surprised. This
is another of society's well-guarded secrets, for whatever reason. Not only
does your relationship with your partner undergo numerous changes, but
having a baby is likely to affect most of your current relationships. Even
if you have an inkling of it beforehand, the enormity of these changes
may shock and alarm you as you struggle to readjust.

Because of all the time and energy you're both devoting to your
child, it's unlikely that you and your partner will have much left over
for each other. This is the normal state of affairs, especially in the first
six to twelve months postpartum. Unfortunately, this abrupt change in
your relationship can lead to problems very fast. Your partner may feel
that the baby is taking all your time, and that he's not getting the attention and affection he needs. You may have similar feelings—you're doing
so much nurturing, yet there's no one around with the time and energy
to nurture *you*.

Perhaps you've gone from spending all your free time together to
having no time alone together after the baby's born. This can lead to resentment, insecurity, and further withdrawal.

Communication will inevitably suffer in this atmosphere of limited
time, physical exhaustion, and growing stress. Your sexual relationship is
likely to change—or disappear altogether—as your patterns of sleeping
and waking change. Your free time is at a premium; when you do have
some time, one or the other of you may just not be interested in making
love. After close physical contact with your baby all day long, and into
the night, the last thing you may want is someone else touching your
body. Your partner has to adjust to your changed body and the fact that

someone else is touching it all the time. If you're nursing, he may feel nervous about your breasts in their new, food-giving capacity. You're different than you were before.

On top of this, you and your partner will need to decide how to divide the child-care responsibilities. This can involve endless jockeying and readjustment, whether it's a question of who changes the soiled diapers or who takes off from work when your child is sick. Even the division of minor responsibilities can lead to conflict—who puts out the garbage, who folds the wash, who does the shopping. If you're on maternity leave, or have quit your job to stay home and raise your child, you may resent the relative ease of your partner's day at work—a day with lunch breaks, quiet time, and adult conversation. Labor laws protect workers from just the sort of job demands you're exposed to every day: endless hours, no breaks. It may seem to you that your partner has no idea what you're going through. At the same time, your partner may feel resentful about working all day and then coming home to a wailing baby, dirty dishes, no dinner, and you looking like the walking dead.

If you both work outside of the home, you may find yourselves scrambling to keep up with your job and care for your new baby. Leaving for work in the morning can become a real marathon as you prepare yourself and your baby for the day ahead. Evenings may be stressful as you and your partner try to unwind from a busy work day and meet your baby's demands. Many working mothers suffer agonies of guilt and anxiety about leaving their child in the hands of other caretakers. This array of emotions and the need to constantly readjust will prove taxing for most couples, and can easily lead to relationship strain.

Remember, infancy doesn't last forever. Gradually, your baby will require less physical care, and you and your partner will have more time for each other. Until then, make an effort to spend time together on a regular basis to nurture your relationship. Talking together even 15 minutes every other night to catch up on the day's events and your state of mind will pave the way for staying in touch. By the time your baby is six months old, once you feel comfortable getting a sitter to fill in for you, we recommend that you and your partner start going out alone together at least every two or three weeks. This will give you a break and renew your relationship, which is, after all, the cornerstone of your family's well-being. It can also be helpful to choose one day a week or every other week during which you get out by yourself and do something you enjoy. Although the stress of having a newborn may not go away, you can follow these suggestions to lessen your stress and preserve your relationship with your partner.

Having a new baby is equally likely to affect, and possibly strain, your relationships with other family members and your friends. Initially, you may find that you have little time or energy for people outside your immediate family. On the other hand, your friends and relatives may be a great source of assistance and emotional support, and you may welcome having them around. Some of your friends and family may not like the choices you make about how you spend your time, and may feel neglected or irritated with the changes in your relationship. Others will be most understanding, and will follow your lead about how you want your relationship with them to evolve, and how they can best support you.

Difficulties may arise from disagreements with your parents or in-laws over how to care for your baby, from the right way to change a diaper to whether it's appropriate to let babies cry themselves to sleep. Some parents and in-laws may be very vocal about their opinions, and you may feel resentful or insecure when they disagree with your child-care decisions. The more your relatives disagree or challenge you, the more angry and/or self-doubting you may become. It's a lucky woman who has supportive parents and in-laws who express their approval about how she's caring for her baby. This approach tends to build confidence, and decrease the fears and insecurity that most new parents have.

In spite of what happens with your family and friends, keep in mind that now is the time to put yourself and your new baby, your partner, and your immediate family first. Think about how much or how little social contact you want, and who you want to spend your time with. Be sensitive to the needs of others, but be most sensitive to your own needs. Listen to what others have to say, and then make your own decisions. Trust yourself to know what is right for you and your new family; and if you change your mind about something, trust in your ability to re-evaluate your options.

18. The Quality of Your Marriage or Partnership

While having a new baby can strain even the best of relationships, you are definitely more at risk for a postpartum reaction if you had problems with your partner before giving birth. Difficulties with communication, spending time together, and expressing affection only intensify with the relationship changes that childbirth brings. Some couples believe that having a child will bring them closer together and solve their relationship problems. This is almost never true. In fact, many troubled relationships end with the added stresses of having a new baby, and this can create a whole new set of problems.

Jeannie was a 36-year-old mother of one who became depressed shortly after her son was born. She and her husband had been married for two years, and were aware of many problems in their relationship. Even before their son's birth, Jeannie's husband felt that he'd given in on several major decisions just to "keep the peace." He admitted in counseling that he'd reluctantly agreed to have a baby because Jeannie wanted one so badly. "I thought that if I didn't go along with what she wanted, our relationship would fall apart. I knew there would be problems, but I didn't think they'd be this great." After the baby's arrival, and all the stresses that came with it, Doug found himself feeling resentful that he had given in. He felt angry rather than sympathetic about Jeannie's postpartum difficulties, because he'd told her that she probably wouldn't be able to handle the stress of having a newborn. Jeannie felt devastated by Doug's lack of support, which only increased her postpartum problems.

Jeannie finally pulled through her depression with counseling and medication; but both she and Doug agree that their marriage almost didn't survive. If they'd had it to do a second time, they would have gotten help well before deciding to have a child.

If there were problems in your relationship prior to your child's birth, you may want to consult a helping professional soon. It's unlikely that things will get better on their own, and they're very likely to get worse. Ultimately, having children can strengthen a couple's bond, if a strong foundation of open communication and caring already exists. But few events tax a relationship as much as the addition of a child. If you are pregnant, or thinking about getting pregnant, and know that your relationship needs help, get it now. Once again, an ounce of prevention is worth a pound of cure. Keep in mind that your relationship with your partner is the cornerstone of your family's well-being. Do not underestimate the importance of this. Get help as you need it to promote your own health and that of your family.

19. The Quality of Your Social Support System

As is the case with problems in your relationship with your partner, you'll have a greater chance of experiencing postpartum difficulties if you lack a strong social support system. By such a system we mean a close network of family and/or friends who provide you with ongoing emotional support, and may offer physical assistance, including helping you care for yourself and your new baby. Having people in your life who care about you, and are there to support you, can be a critical factor in easing postpartum distress. Sometimes just having someone to talk to about how tough things are can be a major relief. By sharing your experiences with family members and friends, you'll discover how common it is for women to go through some emotional upheaval following childbirth, and you'll hear about the ways in which other women have successfully coped with these changes. This knowledge may help you feel less troubled by what you're going through, and more hopeful about what lies ahead. The more you lack social support, the more overwhelmed, frightened, and hopeless you're bound to feel. If you live in an area where other people are not nearby, or have cut yourself off from neighbors and friends, this lack of social support may increase your risk for developing postpartum problems.

Aside from the emotional support that family and friends provide, they may further diminish your postpartum stress by assisting with the physical care of your new baby, and giving you more time to take care of yourself. The more help you get, the quicker your physical and emotional recovery will be. If you have little or no help because of a weak social support system, you're likely to feel more physically and emotionally fatigued, take longer to recover, and be more at risk for developing problems. With little or no opportunity to take a break from your baby's demands and care for yourself, you cannot rebuild your already depleted physical and emotional resources.

If you have a good social support system but are hesitant to ask for help or take the help that's offered, you may also increase your risk of a postpartum reaction. Friends and family may not volunteer to help because they don't want to get in your way; perhaps you haven't let them know you need their help for fear of imposing on them. Maybe you believe that you should be able to do everything by yourself. This is called the superwoman syndrome. Sadly, attitudes can prevent you from getting help you want and need, and that friends and family would gladly give. Take heart—there are steps you can take to stop this from happening.

Before you decide that your friends and family are hesitant or unavailable to help you out, ask them for help with particular tasks and see how they respond. If they show enthusiasm, welcome their assistance. Be specific about what you do and don't need—don't accept babysitting when what you really need is someone to deliver home-cooked food during your first two weeks home from the hospital. Speak up. Stay focussed on your needs. If you're pressuring yourself to do it all, let go of the belief that you possibly can. Instead, practice letting your family and friends share in household and child-care responsibilities, especially in the first few weeks postpartum. By following these suggestions, you can lower your chances of experiencing postpartum difficulties and enhance your postpartum adjustment.

If you have a weak social support system, you may want to think about how to strengthen it. Meeting other new moms can be a big help. Start by finding out what's available in your community. You may be able to join a new moms' group through your local hospital, community college, church, synagogue, or Lamaze class. Many community centers and hospitals offer postpartum health and exercise classes. There may be a playgroup in your neighborhood that other new moms have organized. Look in your community newspaper and on local bulletin boards. When you take your baby out for a stroll, ask other new moms you see what resources they know about. You may learn more through word of mouth than any other resource.

To help you get a break from the physical responsibilities of child care, check again to see what's available in your area. There may be a "Mother's Day Out" program through a local church, where you can drop your baby off for two to three hours once a week for a nominal fee. Usually, you do not have to be a member of the congregation to participate. Your local YWCA or community center may offer babysitting while you take an exercise or crafts class. More recently, licensed play centers have opened where you can drop your child off for a few hours during the week or on the weekend for a charge. This may be particularly helpful for moms who work outside of the home, to get a few hours off on a Saturday or Sunday. Participating in these types of programs may also lead to meeting other parents who may become a source of social support. Form cooperatives with neighbors and friends you make to exchange babysitting and child-care tasks. Help may truly be around the next corner.

20. Being a Single Mom

Being a single mom is another situation that can put you at greater risk for a postpartum reaction. Your risk may be particularly great if you lack a strong social support system and have little or no help caring for your baby. Although this is not characteristic of all single moms, it may be true for many. Very often, single moms find themselves in the position of financially providing for their children, doing all the household chores, and assuming primary care for their children. It's easy to see how such responsibility can lead to increased stress and emotional problems; and it's amazing that so many American women survive this kind of daily existence.

If you became a single mom because of an unplanned pregnancy, this may add to your risk of experiencing postpartum difficulties. Teenagers comprise a large portion of the single mothers in the United States; most of their pregnancies were unplanned. If you are a teenage mom, you're likely to be emotionally unprepared for having a baby—because, in some ways, you may still feel like a child yourself. You may not have the financial means or a family willing to support yourself and your baby; you may need to drop out of school so that you can go to work. You may have an ongoing relationship with your baby's father, or the relationship may have ended, leaving you with the responsibility of raising your child alone. If you're lucky, you at least have your family's support, and can stay with them until you get on your feet. Unfortunately, it may be problems within your family that contributed to your becoming pregnant in the first place. With all that you're going through, postpartum problems may readily occur.

For all single moms of any age, having a strong social support system can ease some of the pressure. If you are lacking such a system, follow the guidelines mentioned in the section on social support. Do what you can to get help caring for your baby. If you can afford it, hire someone to assist you with child-care and household responsibilities. Let friends, family, and neighbors lend a hand as much and as often as they are will-ing. If you're a teenager, look for special resources in your community and through your high school. It may be possible to make arrangements to finish your education or participate in vocational training. There is probably a child-care class in your area especially designed for young mothers, where you and your baby can attend while you learn the physi-cal and emotional skills you'll need for motherhood. Use the resource list at the back of this book to help you locate nearby sources of education and support. Whatever the circumstances of your being a single mom, do what you can to take good care of yourself and your baby. Chapter 5 talks about this topic in greater detail.

21. The Quality of Your Relationship with Your Baby

Aside from your relationship with your partner, family, and friends, the quality of your relationship with your baby can significantly influence your postpartum adjustment. The more difficulties in your relationship with your baby, the more you may be at risk for a postpartum reaction. In most situations, these will be problems that you have not created but are forced to deal with anyway. They include:

- A fussy or "high-need" baby
- A baby with the set of behaviors and symptoms grouped under the general term "colic"
- A baby who must deal with an early childhood illness, injury, birth defect, or disease
- A mismatch in mother-baby temperament

All of these situations can lead to increased stress and tension as you try to develop a relationship with your baby, and can lead to greater self-doubt, frustration, and unhappiness about your new role as a mom.

Although it's not been scientifically proven, there is general agree-ment among parents that some babies are fussier or more difficult than others. Some experts call these "high-need babies." These are babies who tend to be fussy more often or for longer periods of time each day than "easier" babies. Fussy babies may respond less well to your efforts to comfort them, leaving you exhausted, frustrated, and even angry. Some babies require hours of rocking or walking before they'll cry themselves to sleep. If you have such a baby, you may feel constantly drained, both physically and emotionally. Your experience of motherhood so far may feel frustrating and unsatisfying, and this can intensify your postpartum emotional distress. You may wonder how your baby, who appears so per-fect, can be so impossible. You may blame yourself for what is happening, and resent your baby for what he or she is putting you through.

Your pediatrician and other experts may be equally baffled by your baby's fussiness. Experts suggest that as babies grow, and their digestive systems mature, they usually outgrow "colic" or excessive fussiness. If you have not consulted your pediatrician, be certain to do so, so that you can rule out any medical problem. Once you've done this, look at William Sears' book, *The Fussy Baby*, for one expert's practical advice about how to cope.

Make the most of your pleasurable moments with your baby, and take breaks as often as you can to recharge. Enlist all the help with child-care and housework you can find. Most babies respond differently to different caregivers; and you will definitely benefit from a change of pace. Pat yourself on the back for recognizing your limits, and for not putting undue pressure on yourself. Typically, most children outgrow this initial fussiness. Until then, taking good care of yourself will help you have the energy to keep coping.

Colicky Babies

One theory holds that colic results from a lack of development in a baby's digestive system, which can interfere with the baby's ability to smoothly digest breastmilk or formula. Other experts think that colic may be an allergic reaction to the by-products produced when certain types of formula are digested, similar to a lactose intolerance in older children and adults. Regardless of the cause, the symptoms of colic can seriously strain the mother-child relationship. Colicky babies are often most fussy after eating, and may experience visible physical discomfort. You may have difficulty soothing them particularly after mealtimes; it may seem as though there's nothing you can do to help them settle down. You may feel intensely frustrated and angry with your child, extremely incompetent, overwhelmed by feelings of guilt, or some combination of all of the above.

Like fussiness in general, colic appears to subside as your baby matures. Until then, follow the suggestions presented for general fussiness. Some parents have found that running a vacuum cleaner or taking their baby for a drive will help him or her settle down. There are machines and tapes especially designed to create vibrations or "white noise" to soothe colicky babies. Other noise products that may help are stuffed animals that emit a sound similar to a mother's heartbeat, or simulate sounds from within the womb. Everyone will have advice, but you're probably the only person who can figure out what works best for your baby. Remind yourself that it's not your fault that your baby cries all the time. Do what you can to create a positive bond with your baby in spite of the colic. Bonding may take longer, but it will happen.

Serious Medical Problems

If your infant experienced serious medical problems at birth or in the first few months of life, you may feel that you've gone through the emotional wringer. You've probably felt unbearable fear about losing your child. Your sadness and disappointment about what you've had to endure can only be aggravated by your fantasies about what your first few months with your baby would be like. You may be angry at the pain and suffering this has brought on you, your partner, and your child. If you've feared at any time that your child might not live, you may be reluctant to let yourself get too attached. Perhaps you were restricted from holding your baby, or have only limited physical contact because of his or her medical condition. This can also interfere with feeling close. Today, this alienation occurs less frequently, because health-care providers recognize the critical importance of child-parent physical contact and its influence in a sick child's recovery. But if your child has had to stay in the hospital for long periods of time, you will still have been robbed of the sense of closeness and control you'd have in your own home. You or your partner may not be able to spend as much time with your baby as you want to because of your jobs, geographic distance of the hospital, or the needs of your other children. If your baby is at home and requires extensive care, the physical and emotional demands can be overwhelming.

If any of the scenarios above match your own experience, you may be more at risk for a postpartum reaction. Nothing can take away the pain of your child's illness, but talking with friends and family can help. Choosing health-care providers who are understanding and supportive can be equally important. If you don't feel that your child's health-care team is being sensitive to the emotional side of the situation, let them know, or change providers, if you feel you must. Be certain to communicate about what you think is best for you and your baby—such as how much physical contact you'd like, even if it will be difficult to accommodate your wishes because of hospital procedures of mechanical impediments. If your baby is well now, give yourself time to feel safe developing a close and warm relationship. Don't push for sudden changes. Remember, you've been through a lot. The trauma and strain will take time to heal.

Mother-Child Mismatches

Your postpartum adjustment is bound to be affected by the degree to which you and your baby are emotionally alike. Some experts think that the greater the emotional mismatch between mother and child, the greater the difficulty they may have developing a satisfying relationship. This, in turn, may increase your risk for postpartum problems. Perhaps you're quiet and introverted, but your baby is very active, vocal, and outgoing. This sort of mismatch doesn't guarantee a problem, but it may contribute to the difficulty of your postpartum adjustment. Just as adults with different personality types may find it difficult to live together in harmony, you may experience similar personality clashes with your baby.

Instead of viewing your differences as a problem, try to see them as an opportunity for you to explore less obvious aspects of your personality. You may find that, beneath the surface, you're more like your child than you ever could have imagined. If there's simply no way to identify with your baby, then try to think about your child's differences as attributes. You and your baby were one person while you were pregnant. But now your baby is a unique and special person, with strengths and a personality all her own. Help build her self-esteem by valuing who she is and what she has to offer. Don't try to mold her in your own image, but cherish her individuality as much as your own.

22. Your Relationship with Your Other Children

Although having other children has not been identified as a risk factor for postpartum problems, it can influence the quality of your adjustment to your new baby. It all depends on how your children respond to having a new brother or sister, and how their reactions affect you. If your children's response is positive, your adjustment will be easier. Still, it's common to feel some sadness about how caring for your new baby leaves you less time for your other children; you may feel a combination of emotions about how your family has changed. You may feel frustrated and angry with your children's behavior, and guilty and sad about how you have caused it by having a baby. The stronger these feelings become, the more they tend to contribute to postpartum emotional difficulties.

Keep in mind that the upheaval of having a new baby affects the whole family. It will take time for you, your partner, and your children to adjust. Before the baby's arrival, it may be helpful to have your children participate in a sibling class at the hospital where you plan to deliver. At home, encouraging them to talk about their feelings about the baby's upcoming birth, or getting a book on having a new brother or sister, can open the door to later conversations. With younger children, observing their behavior may reveal how they are feeling; you may be able to use their play to deal with some of their uncertainties.

Generally, most children are concerned that the new baby will take your attention and love away from them. And to some extent this is true, especially at the beginning. But you can make a special effort to spend time with your other children on a regular basis after the baby is born. This might mean sharing a nightly bedtime story, or taking a special outing once a week. Try to keep your children's routine as unchanged as possible after the baby comes, to foster a sense of security. Listen to their feelings, but don't feel that you have to make things better overnight. Be realistic with your expectations of your older children, and don't expect them to do more than is appropriate for their age and development. Use discipline as usual. In the face of so much change, caring and consistency will be reassuring to your children, and may improve their postpartum adjustment and yours.

In Summary

Now that you've read about all the risk factors for a postpartum reaction, take a long look at your risk profile questionnaire. Which factors—biological, psychological, or relationship—are affecting you the most? What, if anything, can you do to change them? What assistance can you call on from helping professionals or other resources outside your immediate circle of family and friends?

If you decide to seek outside help, take your completed risk profile questionnaire with you. Give your own assessment of what is going on, and what you think may be needed for things to improve. Use your knowledge of yourself to help your caregiver design the best course of treatment for your particular needs. You can read more about seeking professional help in Chapter 7.

As you work to make changes, refer back to this chapter for advice and suggestions. Take one day at a time. And remember that readjusting to your changed world after having a baby is a tremendous challenge. Be patient but persistent—you *will* get through.

4

Postpartum Survival— Taking Care of Yourself

The Short Version
(If You're Pressed for Time)

It's time now to take stock of exactly what you're feeling, and how much your symptoms—physical or emotional—are getting in the way of how you want to live. This chapter is designed to help you evaluate your feelings and symptoms and develop a plan of action that will help you feel better.

The first step in feeling better is to take care of yourself. The following suggestions can be included in every new mother's (or father's) plan for self-care:

- Take care of yourself physically—get enough rest, eat right, exercise.

- Develop a support system—make sure you have other new parents to talk to, and make a point of talking to them or seeing them at least once a week.

- Express and accept your negative feelings—know that it's normal to feel bad sometimes when you're adjusting to a new baby. You are still an okay person if you don't feel just wonderful about this new addition to your life.

- Attend to your positive feelings—look for ways in which you *do* feel good, and pay attention to these too.

- Take breaks—by yourself, with your partner or another adult. No one can do a job nonstop without some time off every day.

- Keep your expectations realistic—no one can "do it all," let alone do it perfectly. Working toward reasonable, achievable goals, whether having to do with your feelings, the cleanliness of your home, the baby's schedule, control of your body, or whatever other issues are important to you now.

- Nurture your sense of humor—there is great value in keeping in touch with the funny side of life. Try to laugh daily, whether at yourself, your situation, or something outside of all this.

- Structure your day—plan loosely how you will spend your day, with time designated for all the items on this list. Plan for when you will talk to another adult, when you will rest, when you will take a break. Keep the plan flexible and realistic, so that you can stick to it.

- Postpone major life changes—your life is full of enough change and stress right now as it is. Avoid moving to a new job, a new home, a new partner—until you feel more settled in your new role of mother.

Once you have your self-care plan in place, and are working to care for yourself as we have just described, you may begin to feel better. Nonetheless, many of the negative feelings and symptoms that have been plaguing you may not disappear just because you begin to focus on your own needs. The remainder of this chapter is devoted to concrete ideas about what you can do to tackle these problems. You may want to scan the index below. There is advice in this chapter for dealing with each symptom or issue listed below. Place a check mark by each symptom or issue that bothers you. Then, when you have more time, turn to the section addressing that problem, and read more about what might help you feel better. The self-help component of this chapter is divided into three sections: physical symptoms, emotional symptoms, and issues.

Finally, this chapter has a section on getting in gear, putting all the suggestions you've picked out of the chapter to work. For help in finding a peer support group to aid you, contact Depression After Delivery or Postpartum Support International (see the Resources Section at the back of this book).

Exercise
Two Minutes for Yourself

Imagine you have a magic wand. Wave it in the air. What five most pressing things would you change in your life? Write these down in order of importance, listing your highest priority first. Now focus on the top item. Where could you begin to bring about a change in this matter? Think of just one thing you could begin to do *today* that would make a difference. Do that one thing. For example, you may have written "My marriage is falling apart." What would make you feel that things between you and your husband were getting better? Maybe sitting down and talking together for five minutes tonight after the baby is asleep. Talk about something pleasant. Sit close. Remember why you liked each other in the first place. Share some memories about fun times you've shared. Tell each other a secret.

4

Postpartum Survival—
Taking Care of Yourself

Taking Stock

What are your symptoms, and how serious are they? This chapter will help you categorize and weigh the difficulties you're having and will take you step-by-step through the process of making a survival plan. By the time you're done reading this chapter, you'll have a clear idea of what to do to feel better.

We talked about the idea of a continuum, or spectrum, of symptoms in Chapter 2. In the postpartum period, the problems women have don't fit into neat little packages; rather, there's a lot of overlap from one diagnostic category to the next. Women who have the baby blues may cry frequently, but so will women with major postpartum depression.

The chart that follows lists the most common symptoms of postpartum adjustment, organized into three columns representing three bands of increasing seriousness along the continuum. The symptoms are also divided in terms of whether they're mainly physical or emotional, or whether they describe behaviors characteristic of the postpartum adjustment period. Check the box by each symptom that applies to what you've experienced since having your baby. Please keep in mind that the list is only a guide; you may be bothered by symptoms that aren't included here. Write down any additional symptoms in the space provided at the bottom of the chart.

Physical, Emotional, and Behavioral Symptoms of Postpartum Adjustment Problems

Baby Blues/Post-partum Adjustment	Depression/Obsessive-Compulsive Disorder/ Panic (plus the blues)	Psychosis/Mania (plus depression, etc.)
Physical Symptoms		
☐ Insomnia	☐ Headaches	☐ Refusal to eat
☐ Low energy	☐ Changes in sleep patterns	☐ Excessive energy
☐ Appetite loss or food cravings	☐ Hyperventilation	☐ Inability to stop a given activity
☐ Fatigue (even after sleep)	☐ Chest pains	☐ Inability to move
	☐ Heart palpitations	
	☐ Numbness, tingling	
	☐ Shaking, trembling	
	☐ Dizziness, faintness	
	☐ Constipation	
	☐ Diarrhea	
	☐ Itchiness	
Emotional Symptoms		
☐ Anxiety, worry	☐ Despair	☐ Extreme confusion
☐ Extreeme concern over physical changes	☐ Feelings of inadequacy	☐ Loss of memory
☐ Confusion	☐ Inability to cope	☐ Incoherence
☐ Sadness	☐ Feelings of being powerless	☐ Hallucinations
☐ Feeling over-whelmed	☐ Hopelessness	Delusions
☐ Lack of confidence	☐ Extreme concern over baby's health	
	☐ Decreased concentration	
	☐ Loss of normal interests	
	☐ Loss of interest of sex	
	☐ Shame or guilt	
	☐ Suicidal thoughts	

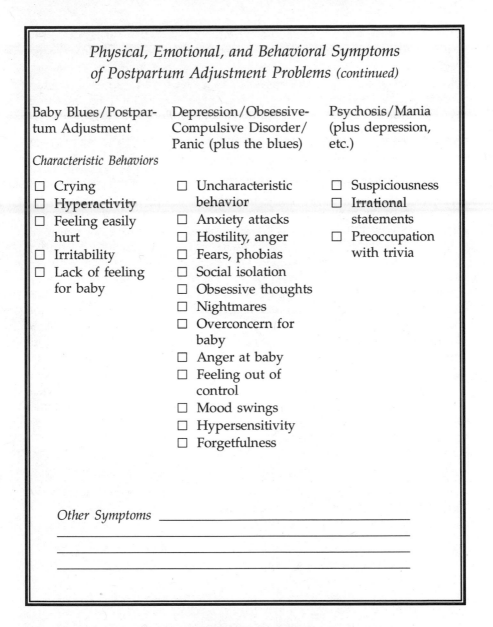

Physical, Emotional, and Behavioral Symptoms of Postpartum Adjustment Problems (continued)

Baby Blues/Postpartum Adjustment	Depression/Obsessive-Compulsive Disorder/Panic (plus the blues)	Psychosis/Mania (plus depression, etc.)
Characteristic Behaviors		
☐ Crying	☐ Uncharacteristic behavior	☐ Suspiciousness
☐ Hyperactivity	☐ Anxiety attacks	☐ Irrational statements
☐ Feeling easily hurt	☐ Hostility, anger	☐ Preoccupation with trivia
☐ Irritability	☐ Fears, phobias	
☐ Lack of feeling for baby	☐ Social isolation	
	☐ Obsessive thoughts	
	☐ Nightmares	
	☐ Overconcern for baby	
	☐ Anger at baby	
	☐ Feeling out of control	
	☐ Mood swings	
	☐ Hypersensitivity	
	☐ Forgetfulness	

Other Symptoms _____

_____

_____

_____

In Case There's a Medical Explanation

You may wonder, "How can I have a postpartum emotional disorder if all my symptoms are physical?" You should call your health-care practitioner and discuss whether there are tests you should be given to rule out general physical causes for your symptoms. Thyroid dysfunction, blood problems, pituitary dysfunction, and even heart problems can cause symptoms similar to postpartum emotional disorders.

Paula was a 33-year-old new mother who felt extremely ill. She couldn't concentrate; she was tired and slept all the time. She was unable to care for her newborn at all, and her sister came to help out. Paula was taken to several doctors to be treated for postpartum depression before she had a complete physical examination that revealed a major heart defect triggered by the stress of childbirth. She underwent open heart surgery and was able to take full charge of her parenting duties in a relatively short time.

Although this sort of case is extremely rare, it does happen. Usually your postpartum checkup will identify a medical problem of this magnitude if one exists. But sometimes women are so caught up with caring for their baby, or feel so overwhelmed by their postpartum adjustment, that they ignore their own medical care. You need to follow through with your checkup even if you were less than satisfied with your care during the birth experience. Find another OB or health professional if you just feel too uncomfortable returning to the person who attended you at your baby's birth. If you're having a lot of physical symptoms apart from those you've been told about, and apart from those that are considered routine, don't wait the usual six weeks for your first postpartum visit. Be sure to return to your caregiver as many times as you need to if symptoms surface after your initial checkup. The small possibility of physical causes unrelated to childbirth needs to be ruled out. It's far more likely that your symptoms have emotional causes. In fact, missing the six-week checkup is considered to be a warning sign of postpartum emotional difficulties.

Getting Help or Helping Yourself

Your postpartum adjustment symptoms may be interfering with your ability to be yourself more than you can tell. A second opinion can help you get the big picture. Ask yourself the following questions, then get a second set of answers from someone you trust.

1. Are you sinking, climbing out of the pool, or treading water? In other words, are things getting worse, better, or staying the same day to day?

2. Do you get showered and dressed more days than not?

3. Do you still do some of the normal things you enjoy doing? (You're not completely stalled by your fears or an inability to "get going.")

4. Are you meeting the baby's needs?

5. Do you feel connected to your baby?

6. Do you feel that your postpartum situation will improve?

If you have only a few symptoms from the chart at the beginning of this chapter, and you answered "yes" to most or all of the questions above, you're probably struggling with a normal postpartum adjustment. Many of the techniques presented in this chapter will be of use to you. If you find that things are getting worse, not better, and you answered "no" to three or more of the questions, you will probably need outside help as well. A professional who is knowledgeable in postpartum difficulties can help you determine your best course of treatment and care. There's information on finding professional help in Chapter 7.

The More You Know, the Better Off You Are

Many women feel relieved when they learn that there's a name for their particular collection of symptoms—when they can say to themselves and others, "This is postpartum depression," or "I am struggling with a difficult postpartum adjustment." Sometimes being able to attach a diagnostic label to your feelings can help legitimize them. It can also take away the feelings of guilt that many new moms feel. The label lets you and everyone else know that you're not just being cranky or weak or spoiled. You're feeling rotten because of specific biochemical changes in your body, and identifiable stressors. There's nothing wrong with you as a person; your hormones are simply out of whack.

Finally, having a label can make it easier to get the help you need. Few health professionals are familiar with the full range of postpartum emotional disorders, but most medical doctors, psychologists, and counselors have at least some understanding of such general terms as *depression* and *obsessive-compulsive disorder*. Being able to apply such terms to your symptoms gives you a kind of power: those you consult will be able to relate to what you're describing, and may be more willing to take your distress seriously.

If you're uncertain about which label best fits your symptoms, go back to Chapter 2, the diagnostic chapter. Read through the descriptions, and use the checklists of symptoms for each postpartum adjustment problem, until you find the label that most nearly describes your own experience.

Taking Care of Yourself

You may have become accustomed to taking good care of yourself physically while you were pregnant. During the first month of your pregnancy, you were probably weighed and examined and given encouragement by your doctor at least once a week. Many women try to eat right, exercise, and get sufficient rest while they're pregnant, spurred on by this attention to their body, and the sense that more than their own health and well-being is on the line.

Once the baby has arrived, though, no one pays much attention to the new mom's body anymore. Apart from your six-week doctor's visit, you're more or less on your own. In fact, people may make a point of not talking about your body, as it's probably looking and feeling a little out of shape right now. All those virtuous habits of self-care go flying out the window. Granted, time constraints and decreased energy make it difficult to keep up (or establish) a routine of exercise, rest, and good eating. Everyone's attention—including yours—shifts to the baby, and it's the baby who gets weighed, measured, and cared for at each doctor's visit now, not you. With the focus no longer on your behavior, it seems much less important. No one fusses over *you*, everyone fusses over the baby—get the message? Besides, taking care of yourself physically is hard work. And it would be selfish, at this point, when your baby needs every minute of your attention, right?

These common misconceptions lay the foundation for many a new mother lapsing into—or even trying to achieve—complete neglect of her own needs in favor of those of the baby. This model of maternal self-sacrifice is rampant in our culture—many of us were raised by mothers who were devoted to this ideal. There's further discussion of this issue in Chapter 9.

Is Your Pitcher Empty or Full?

Take a deep breath, and repeat out loud: "My baby needs a mommy, not a martyr!" Taking care of yourself physically is just as important now as it was when you were pregnant. To be a good mother, first you must be good to yourself, both physically and emotionally. This does not mean, of course, that it's okay to neglect your baby's essential needs for food, warmth, cleanliness, or comfort. But babies are very effective when it comes to making sure that their needs are known. Screaming at 4 a.m., for instance, conveys a pretty clear message, "I need something." What you would be well off aiming for is a balance between your own needs and those of your child. It's best to tackle this issue now, because it's one that you'll be facing for the rest of your life.

A pitcher of water provides a clear demonstration of what we mean. Imagine that you are a pitcher of water. You keep pouring out, and pouring, giving and giving as you take care of the needs of those around you: baby, partner, family, friends. If you do not take action to fill the pitcher up again, pretty soon it will be empty.

No one is a bottomless pitcher. The question is what do you need in order to fill up the pitcher again?

Begin with your physical needs. Continue to take your prenatal vitamins, eat nutritious meals, squeeze in some exercise, get as much rest/sleep/relaxation as you possibly can.

Don't neglect the emotional side of the equation. You truly *need* to talk with others in your same situation, to spend time and share tenderness with your spouse, to have a good laugh, to find at least a small bit of time for activities that gave you pleasure in your pre-baby days. You also need praise—from yourself as well as others—for the job you're doing. Give yourself a pat on the back; ask explicitly for encouragement from your partner, other relatives, the pediatrician, or your friends!

It's impossible to be a good parent to your child if all your own needs go unmet. Give yourself permission to go to the well to refill your pitcher. Value yourself enough to ask others to give you what you need. If the "selfish" label keeps jumping up in your brain, remind yourself that this policy is like insurance or a savings account. You might prefer to use the money (or energy) now on something else, but down the road you'll be glad you invested (in yourself) for your child.

A further benefit of taking care of your own needs is the signal that you give to others. When you take care of yourself, other people treat you—and your needs—with respect. If you have a daughter, you will be providing her with a healthier role model than that of the self-sacrificing mother. If you have a son, you'll be giving him a valuable lesson about the way in which women should be treated and valued (your future daughter-in-law will thank you!).

The rest of this chapter is devoted to the ways in which you can keep your pitcher filled—so that you can be the sort of giving person you want to be.

Making a Survival Plan

The Basics

Every new mother needs to establish the habit of taking care of herself during the hectic days, weeks, and months following the birth of her baby. The groundwork for your survival plan should include the following elements. You need to:

- Nurture yourself physically
- Develop a support system
- Express and accept negative feelings, while also attending to positive feelings
- Take breaks
- Keep your expectations realistic
- Nurture your sense of humor
- Structure your day

- Postpone major life changes

These elements are all discussed in detail below.

Nurture yourself physically. It's absolutely essential to your physical and mental health that you take care of your physical needs. You need to get adequate sleep and rest. You need to eat properly; vitamin supplements are important, but they're not a cure for loading up on junk food. The U.S. Department of Agriculture has revised their recommendations on nutrition recently, changing from a concept of the four food groups to the "Food Pyramid." The pyramid is shown below.

Physical exercise is the third leg of this basic foundation. The benefits of aerobic exercise are well-known for losing those unwanted pounds and toning up. Increasing your activity level with exercise can also provide great stress relief as well as raise your spirits. Look for a postpartum exercise class where babies are welcome. Talking with other moms with babies provides the added benefit of social support. Having this support is a real hedge against negative feelings.

Food Guide Pyramid

A Guide to Daily Food Choices

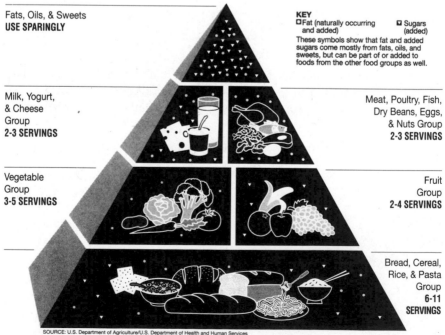

Fats, Oils, & Sweets
USE SPARINGLY

KEY
☐ Fat (naturally occurring   ◪ Sugars
and added)   (added)
These symbols show that fat and added sugars come mostly from fats, oils, and sweets, but can be part of or added to foods from the other food groups as well.

Milk, Yogurt,
& Cheese
Group
2-3 SERVINGS

Meat, Poultry, Fish,
Dry Beans, Eggs,
& Nuts Group
2-3 SERVINGS

Vegetable
Group
3-5 SERVINGS

Fruit
Group
2-4 SERVINGS

Bread, Cereal,
Rice, & Pasta
Group
**6-11
SERVINGS**

SOURCE: U.S. Department of Agriculture/U.S. Department of Health and Human Services

Develop a support system.   Getting together with other parents, who share similar concerns and needs, has been shown to prevent postpartum depression. Just seeing other moms struggling with the same problems you're grappling with can be validating. It's not that misery loves company, but rather that you may no longer feel as if something is wrong with you when you hear another human being voice your feelings, worries, complaints, and concerns.

There are additional benefits to knowing other parents with babies. You may learn new ways of doing things, or about resources for you and your child. You may be able to share something valuable that *you've* learned. There's also the possibility of babysitting trade-offs. You may feel more comfortable leaving your baby with a parent whom you've watched care for her own child than with a babysitter or in a daycare situation. Spending time with other moms, it's relatively easy to judge who sticks to the same standards you do. Especially if you're nervous about leaving your baby with someone else, this may be the most comfortable way—for both of you—to begin. Besides that, it's affordable!

Aside from the benefits of babysitting and validation, socializing with other new parents means that you and your spouse can see how other couples deal with the stresses and strains of adjusting to parenthood. Seeing your own anxious bickering played out by others can give you an entirely new take on your problems. It can be a great relief as well to see that you're not the only couple falling apart at the seams. Your partner can get a chance to relate to other new dads.

Express and accept negative feelings, while also attending to positive feelings.   It takes a great deal of emotional energy to avoid thinking about the hard part of this life change. The harder you work to push those scary or depressing feelings away, the less time and energy you have to live your life. If you can allow yourself to voice your negative feelings somewhere safe, you may find yourself free to experience the positive aspects of having a new baby as well. Writing your feelings out in a diary or journal, talking them into a tape recorder, or expressing them to your partner, a family member, or trusted friend can help you move on. Again, meeting with other new parents may make it easier to do this, as those in the same boat will often understand more easily. Setting aside a time each day to feel and review your feelings can be helpful. You might need to set a timer to remind yourself to switch gears. After your "thinking time," do some deep breathing or stretching, and make a list of your positive feelings.

Take breaks.   How can you expect to fill up that pitcher again if you never get a few minutes off duty? Breaks are the law in the paid working world. They should be in your daily life as well. You need a few minutes to read the paper, sip some tea, put your feet up and just dream. You also need an hour or two away to do something fun. The new mother needs breaks alone, and the couple needs breaks from life as "just parents." This is a very important way to nurture your relationship with your partner, and for you each to nurture yourselves as individuals.

Keep your expectations realistic. If you had grand ideas about reading the complete works of Shakespeare or wallpapering all the bedrooms while you were home on maternity leave, recognize these notions for what they are: completely unrealistic fantasies. The day-to-day care of a new baby is physically demanding and time-consuming to an incredible degree. If you get to *shower* every day you'll be doing well.

Here are two things you can do to help you keep your expectations in line with reality. First of all, keep a list for a day or two of every baby-care task you complete. Run a tally of the number of times you change the baby, feed the baby, wipe up the spit-up, wash the clothes, rock the baby, walk the baby, write a thank-you note, bathe the baby. At the end of a couple of days, you'll be amazed at how much you're accomplishing—even though these particular tasks might not have been exactly what you had in mind when you were building your castles in the sky. Nonetheless, all of these tasks are essential; hiring a baby nurse to do them would cost a great deal of money. Secondly, if you must make a "to do" list beyond infant care, make it only two items long. If you accomplish one of these tasks, you're batting 500. Most professional baseball players would be thrilled with such a performance. Pat yourself on the back. You deserve it.

Nurture your sense of humor. The ability to step back and see the absurdity and/or hilarity in a situation is *always* a valuable asset. This is especially critical when you have a new baby around. If you're having trouble seeing anything funny about your days, take a deep breath, sit back, and exhale slowly. Try to imagine looking back on this scene two or three or even ten years from now. Think about your funniest stories from other times in your life. Chances are they revolve around a minor disaster of one kind or another. Believe it or not, some of your worst days now will make great stories later on.

Judy had two babies in 13 months, leaving her with her hands full. The second baby was a real "spitter," regurgitating after feedings so often that Judy became concerned and called the pediatrician. She was tired of needing to wear white every day and smelling like a cheese factory. The doctor asked her to tally how many times the baby spit up each day. She got to 147 before 3 p.m. one day before giving up! While this drove her to tears at the time, it made a hilarious story by the time the baby turned one. (He was fine even in the midst of his spitting, gaining weight like crazy.)

Imagine what might seem funny about your own scenario three years from now. If you're having difficulty, check out some of Bill Cosby's or Robin Williams' comedy routines about parenthood from the video store. Or look in the library or your book store for *Baby Blues* by Rick Kirkman and Jerry Scott.

Besides trying to keep focused on the humor in your daily chaos, look for other ways to inject some levity into your life. Read the comics. Listen to comedy routines on radio or tape. Watch a funny TV program. Check out a joke book from the library. Look at old childhood pictures, or call up some old childhood friends. Figure out what works best to tickle your funny bone, then take five minutes each day to nurture your sense of humor. It pays off in a better mood and an increased amount of energy.

Structure your day.   The night before, while you're still thinking clearly, sit down and plan out your agenda for the next day. It helps to have at least one outing to look forward to each day—even if it's just a walk around the block. If you feel anxious about going out, schedule a telephone call to a friend. Try to plan at least one event involving adult contact, beyond your partner's return in the evening. Plan for something fun, too, even something as simple as reading the comics or watching a TV show you enjoy. Such planning is an important way to regain a sense of control in your life, even if you're only controlling a few small events every day.

Postpone major life changes.   The first several months postpartum are no time to decide anything that will have long-term consequences. Do not move, change jobs, file for divorce, or make any other big decisions unless you have absolutely no other choice. You'll be much better equipped to tackle such issues when your hormones are back in balance, and you've begun to adjust to your new life as a mom. Dads are also well-advised to resist the urge to turn their lives any more upside-down than they are already.

If you can put all these recommendations to work in your life, a little bit at a time, you may begin to feel a lot better. No one can do all of these things perfectly, or do them 100 percent of the time. But taking charge in these few, but major, areas can get you back on the road to feeling like yourself again. This is the basic foundation for your survival plan.

We know from experience that some problems require a more specific plan of action. After you've given the recommendations above your best shot, read our suggestions below for dealing with the other common complaints and symptoms. Scan the whole index first, and make check marks by the relevant symptoms. Then go back and read one group of suggestions at a time. Give yourself the chance to absorb these ideas in a leisurely fashion—there's no quick fix for postpartum adjustment problems, and you won't be able to address all your symptoms at once. Just deal with one item at a time—maybe one item a day. Then see if you feel better after a week of making minor positive adjustments to your routine.

How To Cope with Particular Symptoms

Thirty years ago, women spent at least a week in the hospital after having a baby. But over time, expectations and insurance regulations have changed. New mothers are no longer given much time at all to recover, either in the hospital or at home. Sometimes it helps to have explicit permission to take care of yourself physically. You may need to plan your day to include naps, exercise, and physical pampering. Soaking in the bathtub or treating yourself to a massage, professional or otherwise, can be extremely comforting. Your diet is important, especially those vitamins and minerals that are depleted by pregnancy, childbirth, and lactation. Taking care of yourself physically is one way to say, "I'm important—my health matters."

Before you head into our descriptions of specific symptoms and solutions, make sure you've read and worked on the basic foundation described earlier. It's almost impossible to relieve particular symptoms if you're not getting adequate rest, nutrition, and emotional nurturing. Add the suggestions listed here only after your primary needs are being addressed. Any persistent physical symptoms should be checked out by your health-care provider to rule out an underlying medical problem. If you've been given a clean bill of health, and still have symptoms, try some of the ideas from the list below.

Physical Symptoms

Low energy and fatigue.   The lack of energy and extreme fatigue felt by many new mothers is due in large part to sleep deprivation and hormonal imbalances. You probably won't feel fully restored until a certain amount of time passes postpartum—how much time depends on your physical condition and the nature of your birth experience. But certain measures *can* help.

The old advice to sleep when your baby sleeps is still good advice, even though it can be hard to follow. If you can't sleep, at least designate a rest period of 20 minutes or so to put your feet up with a tall glass of water, juice, or herbal tea within easy reach. Listen to music or read something enjoyable. Do not do chores—remember that this is your official break time. If your baby doesn't sleep sufficiently during the day to allow you to rest, call on your support network to spell you. Someone else can take the baby out in her carriage, or rock her, while you take a nap or relax.

It may seem illogical, but exercise is also an excellent way to gain more energy. With your weary body, it may take a big push to get yourself moving—but the payoff in energy will be well worth the effort. Walking is probably the best thing you can do now. You can build your endurance gradually, you can take your baby with you, and you'll both get fresh air. If the weather's horrible, see if you can find a gym that has an indoor track, or a mall that allows walkers in before or after store hours. As soon as your OB gives you the okay, swimming is also a great way to regain your strength, although you'll have to get someone else to watch the baby.

Pay attention to your diet, too. If you have a doughnut for breakfast and then feel exhausted by mid-morning, you're probably having a "sugar crash." You need a balanced diet, including low-fat sources of protein. Try to eat lots of fresh fruits and vegetables, and whole grains such as brown rice, oats, and barley. Even if this isn't a diet you're accustomed to, it's one that will keep your system in working order. Snacking on nutritious foods throughout the day—having six small meals—is actually better for you than three full meals, which may be harder to digest.

A fun activity, or good talk with a friend, can also be energizing. If you're running on empty, and not taking some time for yourself, it's no wonder if you feel burned out and tired.

If your fatigue is due to sleep problems read the section below.

Sleep problems.   Sleep problems can take many forms: difficulty falling asleep, either at the start of the evening or after waking to feed the baby; early morning awakening; insomnia; or oversleeping. If you have trouble falling asleep, check out physical causes first. Caffeine (from coffee, soft drinks, tea, or chocolate) is the most common cause. Having a glass of wine or another alcoholic beverage to try to ease yourself into sleep often backfires: the alcohol may relax you at first, but then acts as a stimulant a few hours later. Medications can keep you from sleeping well; talk with your doctor or pharmacist if you suspect that a drug you're taking is disturbing your sleep. Spicy foods or late-night snacks have been known to interfere with dozing off.

If you rule out stimulants, and you're still not sleeping, try to notice what you're thinking about when you lie awake. Anxiety and worry may be the major cause of insomnia in new mothers. See the suggestions later in this chapter for dealing with anxiety.

If you're not getting adequate sleep, you're probably getting more and more worried about how you'll get through your work the following day. Such worry can set up a vicious cycle of worry and sleeplessness. To tackle insomnia, try to follow these guidelines:

- Stick to a regular schedule, especially a waking time. This can help reset your biological clock if it's gone haywire.

- Avoid naps if you're unable to sleep at night. Rest and relax instead.

- Avoid sleep-disruptive drugs and other stimulants such as caffeine.

- Exercise in the morning or early afternoon, but not late in the day.

- Avoid heavy meals or feeling hungry close to bedtime.

- Sleep in a safe, secure, and quiet setting.

- Don't lie in bed for extended periods when you're not intending to sleep. Don't use your bed as a library or an office. Cultivate a strong association in your mind between going to bed and going to sleep.

- Try to wind down and relax in the evening. (This may be difficult if your baby tends to be fussy in the evening. If this is the case, try to get people in your support network to help out in the evening, so that you can get some time to relax.)

- Go to bed only when you're sleepy. (But try to keep to the same schedule every day.)

- If you are not asleep in 10-15 minutes after lying down, go into another room. Do something boring or relaxing—listen to music, read a boring book, listen to a relaxation tape, or imagine a blank screen in your head. Return to bed only when you are sleepy. Again, the goal is to associate bed with falling asleep quickly. Repeat this process if necessary.

- Make it your goal to stay relaxed, rather than focusing on falling asleep. Visual imagery, such as a picture of a restful beach scene, may help you become, and stay, more relaxed.

- To wind down in the evening, try some breathing exercises.

- Have a glass of warm milk or a high carbohydrate snack (such as bread, cereal, bagel, pasta).

- Soak in the bathtub or take a warm shower before going to bed.

- Set your alarm clock but turn the clock around so that you can't watch it.

- Get up at the same time every day.

If your problem is oversleeping—if you can't get up in the morning or you nap all day—a regular sleep schedule will help you as well. Exercise can energize you, as can high-protein snacks. Not being able to get up may be a sign of depression that you cannot easily tackle on your own. If this applies to you, please see the section on seeking professional help.

Appetite or eating changes.   You may find that you suddenly have cravings, or no appetite at all. Keep in mind that a well-balanced diet is essential to your physical and emotional health. Allow yourself reasonable portions of the foods you crave; often, denial of the craved food only makes the craving worse. But try not to binge; and make sure you get adequate portions of all the nutrients you need. If you're nursing, you'll need 300 to 500 extra calories a day—get nutritional advice from your doctor or La Leche League publications, or make an appointment to speak to a professional nutritionist. You'll probably be able to differentiate between cravings for particular foods—tomatoes or sushi, for instance—and an insatiable appetite. If you think you're eating out of emotional need, it may be a good idea to seek professional help (see Chapter 7).

If you have no appetite, work on identifying a few foods that might taste good. "Comfort foods," which you ate happily in childhood or at other times you recall fondly, are a good place to start. Maybe you can eat small amounts of soup, for instance, gradually adding bread or fruit to broaden your diet. If you find that you cannot force yourself to eat, or you're throwing up after you eat, get professional help right away.

Hyperactivity.   Perhaps you feel driven to accomplish everything. You can't stop and rest; you feel very jumpy inside. If you can, force yourself to take rest times, breathe deeply, and reduce the number of things you are trying to accomplish. Make sure you are exercising. Watch your intake of caffeine and sugar; both of these substances can "hype" you up. If you cannot make yourself slow down, you must seek professional help. You may be experiencing postpartum mania, and may be at risk for a more serious postpartum adjustment problem.

Panic symptoms.   Hyperventilation, dizziness, shaking, hot or cold flashes, numbness or tingling, and heart palpitations can all be signs of a panic attack. Panic attacks are triggered by biological changes, and can be treated medically. Please see the section later on *anxiety, worry, or obsessive thoughts*.

Stomach pain or butterflies.   Feeling fluttery or achey in your stomach has been associated with postpartum obsessive-compulsive disorder. See the section later on *anxiety, worry, or obsessive thoughts*.

Constipation or diarrhea.   Exercise and proper diet are essential in maintaining proper bowel function. The soreness from childbirth, hemorrhoids from pregnancy, and little time to oneself can contribute to problems in this area. You may need to get on a schedule, allowing yourself quiet time at home to relax. Take time for yourself alone in the bathroom at this time, even if the baby needs to be put in the swing or the crib for a few minutes alone. Anxiety can also contribute to constipation or diarrhea. See the section later on *anxiety, worry, or obsessive thoughts*.

Itchiness. Dry skin can result from hormonal changes. Pamper yourself with some nice lotion; have your partner rub some soothing cream on your back, or soak in a bathtub with baby oil added. Itchiness can also be a sign of emotional turmoil, so pay attention to your feelings and read the relevant sections that follow.

Headaches or spots before the eyes. Headaches and seeing spots or halos can be signs of stress, anxiety, and depression—although you want to be sure to rule out an underlying medical problem before making this assumption. Read the relevant sections that follow, and make sure you get some exercise and adequate time to relax every day. Migraine headaches can be particularly debilitating, but in recent years have been managed through medication, biofeedback, Chinese medicine, and other alternative approaches. Find out what resources are available in your area—look for practitioners who have a record of success.

Physical tension, stiff and sore muscles. Without doubt, the hard work of labor and birth can leave you feeling stiff and sore. Gentle exercise and pampering are the key to relieving tension and soreness. Be sure to always warm up before you exercise by bending and stretching. Make the time to have a relaxing bath or massage.

Your feelings can also add to tension and actual physical soreness in your body. If you are stiff and sore long after the birth, but feel fine emotionally, have a thorough medical evaluation to look for causes. You may also want to consult a chiropractor or posture specialist about the proper way to lift, nurse, and carry your baby to minimize muscle strain. Pay attention to your body. It may be trying to tell you to take it easy.

Emotional Symptoms

Crying. Crying and tearfulness in the postpartum period can have any number of causes. Tears can come from feeling overwhelmed, tired, frustrated, depleted, hungry, or sleepy. You may feel a sense of loss about any number of issues: your life as it was before the baby came; the contrast between your dreams of the perfect baby or delivery, and the way things turned out; your figure and how long it's taking you to lose the weight you gained during pregnancy; and so on. Use the suggestions in this chapter for addressing each of these underlying causes: read the recommendations for *sleep problems, loss, and trouble coping.*

If none of these issues seems to strike a chord for you, and/or you just feel like crying, go ahead and cry. Crying can be beneficial in releasing stress. Set aside 15 or 20 minutes each day to cry out your feelings. Set the kitchen timer, collect the tissues, and cry. Or cry in the shower. If you fear you will not be able to stop once you begin, setting the timer or an alarm clock, and planning an activity (exercise, a shower) for when your crying session ends, can enable you to take control. If you find that you cannot truly control the crying in this way, see the section on getting professional help.

Confusion or trouble with concentration.   It's common in the postpartum period for new mothers to feel "muddled." You may lose your train of thought, forget what you were going to say or do, or even become confused about what day of the week it is. This muddled state of mind is likely caused by a combination of fatigue, concentration on the new job of being a parent, and fluctuating hormones. To remedy this, first make sure that your habits for rest, relaxation, and diet are in good shape. Try to decrease overload and expectations—having fewer jobs to keep track of will help. Make lists and write things down, but keep your lists simple. Many women find it most useful to make their (brief) lists the night before, rather than in the morning when they're feeling groggy. Pick your most alert time, and plan your day then. Using a calendar with reminders, and checking off each day, can orient you about the passage of time. Take rest breaks, when you close your eyes briefly, using your imagination like a TV screen to focus on important tasks or items to remember. If your partner or family members are more organized than you're feeling now, let them call you or write you notes with daily reminders. (But avoid this if their reminders feel more like pressure than help—stay attuned to what works for *you*.) Talking to yourself, naming the task at hand or item to remember, can help you stay focused. If you forget what you went to the baby's room for, recite it to yourself while you're walking there the next time. "I am going to get the blanket, I am going to get the blanket," may feel strange at first, but it will put you back in control. If feelings are getting in the way and interfering with your concentration, attend to those feelings. (See the relevant entries that follow: *Anxiety, worry, and obsessive thoughts; sadness or hopelessness; loss* (in the issues section); *lack of confidence, feelings of inadequacy; or trouble coping, feeling overwhelmed or powerless.*

Trouble coping, feeling overwhelmed or powerless.   Everything may be feeling as if it's crashing in on you. You can't get anything done; you feel as if you have little or no control over the day's events and your reactions to them.

First of all, single out one area in which you do have control, and in which you are accomplishing something. This may be as simple as getting the baby's diaper changed when needed. You *are* succeeding here. Write this down on a notecard and post it somewhere: "I am getting the baby's diapers changed every day." Pat yourself on the back. Reassure yourself that there is nothing wrong with you for feeling overwhelmed with your life. Adjusting to a new baby and accomplishing all the work involved *is* a mammoth task. You do have control in some areas—exercise that control. Make the bed every day, or clean one room and keep that one room clean. Decide on one task you will do per day and get that one task done. Slowly add one more task at a time, never adding more than you can reasonably hope to accomplish. Sit down with your partner or a trusted friend or family member and examine your expectations. Throw out any expectations that are unrealistic. Brainstorm about ways to get help getting basic chores done—things that will make your life miserable if they're left undone. Can you afford to hire someone to help clean your house? Is there someone in your support network who will shop for you until you're able to handle the shopping? Can you and your husband eat nutritious take-out food a few times a week to cut down on the cooking and shopping until you're feeling well? Can you lower your housekeeping standards until you have more time? Take things one day at a time, and focus on the tasks you manage to accomplish—not on everything that's still not done. Keep in mind that the chaos in your life now is temporary.

Lack of confidence, feelings of inadequacy.   Few people feel like a parent when they take home that new baby. If you find yourself saying, "Where did this baby come from, and what am I supposed to do with him?" you are completely normal. It's a myth that you will suddenly *know* what your baby needs or what to do to feel like a parent. Reassure yourself, your partner, your baby, and your family (if they are asking) that you certainly can learn to fulfill your role as a parent. What is important is that *you* know you can, and that you tell yourself this. Write it down and post it on notes around the house if you need reassurance: "I can be a good enough parent." "I can be a person and a parent, too." Read these affirmations to yourself at various times throughout the day. Do some research if this will reassure you. Talk to friends or relatives about their parenting styles, scan some books, watch parenting shows on TV, and find out what feels right to you. There are a myriad of styles and answers to parenting questions. Give yourself permission to find a style that suits you, and to take as much time as you need to develop. Good parenting is a process, not an exact science. What works for one child and one family may not work for another. There is no *one* right way. Take a parenting course if this will boost your confidence, or call a parent information hotline if you need specific answers right now. And keep telling yourself, "I can do this."

Sadness or hopelessness.   Feelings of sadness tend to well up easily in the postpartum period. This might seem strange to you in the context of everyone saying, "Lucky you—this is the happiest time of your life!" Expectations that your life *should* be wonderful now only make you feel worse, making you wonder, "What's the matter with me?" In reality, it's not uncommon to feel sad when you have a new baby. If you can identify some of the reasons underlying your sadness, list them on a piece of paper or talk about them with your partner or a trusted friend. Allow yourself to feel sad, and ask others to reinforce this permission, telling you it's okay to feel your feelings. If you can pinpoint specific causes, evaluate whether there are problems that can be solved, or whether there's a situation you will need to grieve. If your unhappiness stems from something that's changeable, define the change you'd like to see, and make a plan for moving toward that goal. If you're dealing with a condition—something that's subject to change, see the entry on *loss* in the issues section.

Hopelessness is a sign that should not be ignored. If you have identified causes, work to take control of the parts you can change. See the entry earlier on *trouble coping, feeling overwhelmed or powerless*. If you feel unable to tackle your feelings of hopelessness, see Chapter 7 on getting professional help.

Irritability or hypersensitivity.   Fluctuating hormones, fatigue, and the uncertainties that go with being a new parent are all big contributors to the irritability and hypersensitivity that new mothers often feel. Take a look at when your feelings get hurt most quickly, and see if any patterns exist. Does it happen when you are tired, or hungry, or when you've been alone all day? Is it worst in the evening, when you are looking forward to your partner's return, and your expectations of "relief" are high? If you can see factors that trigger your irritability, work to change them. If your partner wants to come home and play with the baby, leaving you feeling neglected, speak up. Give yourself permission to ask for some attention, too. If you're feeling overwhelmed, see the earlier entry on *trouble coping, feeling overwhelmed or powerless*. Often it helps to write down your feelings, in a journal or letter. Having an outlet for negative feelings makes them less powerful. Clear communication can take away some of the hurt. If you feel that someone is criticizing your behavior, go ahead and ask them to reword their statement. If your spouse comes in at the end of the day and says, "You're still in your nightgown!", it might sound like he's saying, "What did you *do* all day?" Asking him to clarify what he means might reveal that he really wanted to say, "You poor dear—was it rough today?" If he *was* taking you to task for not getting dressed, let him know more of the details of your day so that he can develop a little more empathy. Tell him clearly that you don't have any tolerance for criticism now—you're feeling insecure enough as it is. Tell him and others around you that you need to hear supportive statements and encouragement for the time being.

Taking several deep breaths and counting to ten are old standbys for preventing an all-out fight being triggered. When you give yourself time to think through what bothered you about another person's comment, you can evaluate whether your perceptions are accurate and fair, and you may be able to respond in a more measured and reasonable way. Some people are simply toxic in the amount of criticism they deal out, or in the way they play on your insecurities. It may be necessary to steer clear of these people while you're in such a vulnerable state, no matter who they are—whether your mother, your sister-in-law, or your nearest neighbor. If it's your partner who's pressing your buttons, try to convince him to enter couples therapy with you.

A lack of feelings toward the baby, anger, or overprotectiveness. The idea that bonding takes place on the delivery bed is an old myth that dies hard. The attachment process is a slow, gradual growth of feeling between you and your baby. As you get to know your child, you will feel stronger feelings—and all of these feelings may not be positive. Feeling angry or overprotective toward your baby may occur as you become attached for many reasons. You may spend more time with the baby than with any other person. The baby may be the source of most of your joy as well as your frustration with your life right now. After all, you did not feel this way before the baby appeared. Read the entries below on *worry, anxiety, or obsessive thoughts*; and the entry on *anger* in the issues section later.

Worry, anxiety, or obsessive thoughts.   You may find that you are "stuck" on certain worries or thoughts that make you feel anxious. Anxiety and worry frequently plague new parents. Surviving pregnancy and childbirth may give you a new awareness of the fragile nature of human life. You see how small and vulnerable your baby seems. And you are inclined to protect him or her. Seeing how small babies are, and then comparing them to the world of violence and potential harm we live in, it is quite natural to wonder (and worry) about how they'll ever grow to reach adulthood. And then for you to be in charge of that—how overwhelming! It's in this reasoning process that worries tend to surface.

You can't protect your child from every danger in the world. But not all those threats come barging in the door at once, either. You'll have time to teach your child as best you can to live as wisely and safely as possible. In the meantime it's your job to protect your baby the best *you* can for the next few years.

Nonetheless, many events that affect your child are simply not subject to your control. You can't control weather or wars or an uneven pavement that may cause your child to trip and fall. You can't shield your child from every disease-bearing cough or sneeze or handshake. To manage your worries and anxieties, you can first make sure you're taking all the recommended steps to care for your child. Use a car seat, get those vaccinations, feed her well, make sure no one smokes in your household. For your own peace of mind, you may want to quit reading the newspaper or watching the evening news or talk shows for a while. It can be helpful to have a "worry time" set aside each day. Keep a tablet close by throughout the day. When worries surface, jot them down and tell yourself, "I'll think about that later, during my worry time." When the appointed time arrives, get out the tablet and focus on it for 20 or 30 minutes, really allowing yourself to worry and think about possible precautions. When the time is up, switch gears with a distracting activity (exercise, pampering) and begin to put aside your worries for the next session. You'll free up much of your energy through the day by saving the worries for one set time. Writing worries on an erasable board and symbolically "erasing" them at the appointed time can help put them out of your head. Talk your worries into a tape recorder or to your partner. Drawing them and then tearing them up may relieve you as well. Wearing a fat rubber band on your wrist and snapping it, saying "stop" when you cannot get a worry out of your head, can also help you switch gears. Or close your eyes and picture the concern on a screen in your head. Then change channels to an image of a relaxing or positive scene, or a blank screen.

Obsessive thoughts are those thoughts or ideas that occur again and again. A new mother will often feel as if these thoughts come from "nowhere," and that she's unable to control or stop them. If you have repetitive thoughts, and the suggestions you've read here offer little relief, please seek professional help. You may have an obsessive-compulsive disorder, which is biologically caused and can be cured with medication. Refer to Chapter 7.

Issues

Symptoms, as described earlier, are actual physical, emotional, and behavioral experiences you may have in the postpartum period. Issues, on the other hand, are the underlying concerns that may lead to those symptoms. You cannot formulate a survival plan that just works to relieve the symptoms. Rather, most new mothers need to pay attention to the feelings and changes required of them as they adjust to this new baby (whether their first or their fifth). This section can help you identify and sort out the major effects the birth of this child has had on your life.

Social support or social withdrawal.   Whether you know and talk often with other people who have babies can make a big difference in your life postpartum. Research has shown that those new parents who talk regularly with a person who understands their trials and joys have an easier adjustment than do new parents without such friends. But making new friends, or time for the ones you do have, can seem impossible when you have a new baby and can barely get yourself dressed each day. Making friends as an adult isn't as easy as it was in childhood or college days, when there was a ready supply of prospects at school, and you may have felt more open emotionally, and more willing to take risks. You may have few women who stay at home on your block, or no co-workers with children. If you need to find potential friends, getting out and approaching other mothers you see is essential. Speak to them in the grocery store or the park. Advertise at your pediatrician's office or your church. Take a postpartum exercise class, or a mom-baby class, at your local recreation center. Check with your local mental health association about new mother groups in your area (look in the city or county listings in your phone book under "Mental Health Association").

Once you have spotted a person or two who is in the same boat, make getting to know that person a priority. Or, if you already know someone, commit to meet with her on a regular basis. Plan a coffee break, start a play group or a babysitting co-op, schedule a daily walk or take an exercise class together. Even planning a daily talk on the phone with friends can provide a much-needed opportunity to compare notes, commiserate, and share solutions. You may have to work on keeping in touch with friends this way. Think of it as another habit you want to develop in your determination to take care of yourself.

Control and perfectionism.   These may seem like two very different issues, but in practice they're intimately related. Control is a matter of wanting everything to be "the right way," which often translates into 1) wanting things to be perfect, and 2) wanting things to be *your* way. When you have a new baby, it's often difficult to accept the many aspects of your life that you can't control. Your life may no longer seem perfect, or as nearly perfect as it was before. You can't make the baby sleep. You can't make yourself sleep at times. Often, you can't make the baby stop crying. You can't control what your partner does or says; he may not be the perfect parent you hoped he'd be. Your formerly lovely house may be a total mess, with laundry and baby things and dirty dishes and wilted flowers everywhere. This all may make you feel extremely out of control, as if you can influence nothing in your life.

Perhaps you've been accustomed to controlling your life to a great extent. You may have finished your education, delaying marriage and having a baby until the time was right. This may mean that you'd finally bought a home, or planned the baby for a certain time of year, or had saved enough money so that you could stay home with the baby for several years. The cold, cruel reality of not being able to control your life to this extent anymore may now be hitting you hard. It may be time to adjust your expectations; time to identify those issues that you *can* control in your life right now. You have to choose your battles from now on. Some things may just have to be let go so that you can relax and enjoy life more. You can't control the baby and her schedule, any more than you can make your partner do things your way. Often, making a conscious decision to let go and not control everything (a futile goal, anyway) can be helpful. Tell yourself, "I can't make everything perfect," or "I need to let go of what I can't change." Give yourself permission to no longer be the one in charge of everything and everybody.

You may need to push yourself to make mistakes in order to have a chance to accept them. You will not know that mistakes and imperfection are tolerable, and not life-threatening, unless you actually make them.

Experiment with some little things. Put the baby's shirt on backwards or inside-out. If you are picking up the toys (or clothes or books and papers) every time the baby goes to sleep, practice leaving them out instead. Don't wear make-up one day. Serve cereal for dinner. All of these small imperfections can broaden your perspective. You goofed, and life went on. Pick some mistakes you can tolerate, and work your way up to bigger ones. (However, don't lose sight of things that are critical. You still need to pay bills on time, drive the speed limit, and change the baby's diaper when it's soiled.)

While you are working on making little mistakes, pay attention to what goes on in your head. Your thinking is really a matter of talking to yourself: psychologists call this "self-talk." What you say to yourself influences the way you feel. You'll feel better if your self-talk is positive, rather than negative or "toxic." Remind yourself that you are being a "good-enough" parent or partner. Make up some positive affirmations— "I am a worthwhile person who sometimes makes mistakes," "I'm a loving mother, and I'm doing the best I can right now"—and write them on notecards or self-adhesive note pads. Post your notes on your mirror, above the changing table, on your dashboard, or on the refrigerator door. When you read them, practice thinking about yourself in a different way. You can do things imperfectly, and leave some things undone, and still be an immensely valuable person. That baby of yours doesn't care if the bed is made or the towels match.

You may want to refer back to the entry on *trouble coping, feeling overwhelmed or powerless* for more ideas on changing your perspective.

Anger.   Anger may be the feeling that you least expected to have after the birth of your baby. What on earth do you have to feel angry about, you may ask yourself. You may even be asked that question by others. Rest assured that anger is a common postpartum emotion for many women, and it may seem incredibly strong.

There are legitimate reasons to be angry after having a baby. Most of them have to do with expectations. You did not expect to feel so badly. You did not expect to feel so out-of-control. You did not expect your baby to cry all the time, or be a boy, or girl, or look like your father, or be sick, or colicky, or any number of other things that have come to pass. You did not expect to have the birth experience you had. You did not expect to feel neglected by your partner, parent, friend, etc. You expected your loved ones to be more helpful and involved. You expected to get some rest, and to look and feel better sooner. You may feel cheated about any number of things. And while you may be surprised about having these feelings, there's nothing wrong with you for feeling them. You are not crazy.

However, you may need to adjust your expectations a bit. Refer back to the entries on *trouble coping, feeling overwhelmed or powerless,* and in this section *control and perfectionism.* The entries that follow on *dysfunctional family of origin, uninvolved or absent partner, loss,* and *relationship difficulties* may be helpful. Chapter 9 of this book looks at the problem of expectations in general, working toward a model that is more supportive of women. You may need to find a safe outlet for your anger. If you push your anger down inside you, and deny or minimize its importance, it's more likely to explode over some minor hurt or insult. Such an explosion can blow everything out of proportion, and may also make you feel as though you've lost your credibility as a reasonable person. It may also make you feel uncomfortably out of control.

Try getting your anger out in some physical way. Exercise, jump rope, punch a pillow, throw or kick a ball, break eggs in the sink, blow up a paper bag and pop it. Take a shower and scream in the shower, or scream in your car with all the windows rolled up. Or scream silently: clench your fists, tense your shoulders, prepare to scream but let only the air, not the noise, out of your mouth. You may find relief in writing out your feelings in a journal or scribbling them on paper. Tearing paper or phone books can relieve lots of anger and tension. Make ugly, angry faces in the mirror. Go out in the backyard and stomp around. Make a list of what anger activities work for you and keep it handy, so that you can easily pick one when you feel about to explode. If anger is a problem for you, try to do some of the things on the list every day, even before you feel about to explode. Consider it insurance.

Speaking up is also an important way to diffuse anger. Keep in mind that you want your expression of angry feelings to be assertive, not aggressive. You want to speak your mind without hurting others. Use the word "I" rather than "you." Avoid name-calling or accusations. Stick to the event at hand, rather than the last 40 anger-provoking events in your life. For example, say, "I was angry when you walked in and right past me to the baby. I want you to greet me first." This will get you to a solution much quicker than saying, "You are so heartless—you ignore me all the time." Try to be specific about what was done, and what you would like to have done differently. And realize that you have a right to express your angry feelings, but so does the other person. Be prepared to listen, and to acknowledge the other person's feelings. "I didn't know you were angry, too," can go a long way toward soothing someone's feelings. Finally, expressing your anger may not accomplish anything more than making you feel better by getting the anger off your chest. Keep your expectations in check here, too. Remember that you're expressing your anger as a way to make yourself feel better. You're not getting your anger out to make someone else feel guilty, or as a way to control someone. Change *may* come about as a result of your words, but there are no guarantees.

Dysfunctional family of origin.   Perhaps in your family of origin your feelings were not respected, or you were not allowed to be yourself.

You may feel a deep hurt about wrongs inflicted on you by your family. Your parents may have provided models that you desperately don't want to copy; you may fear imposing their parenting style on your own child. There are many ways in which the family in which you grew up can influence your own transition to parenthood, and you may feel a need to face those family issues once your own baby has arrived.

You may need to do some serious thinking about what needs to be different. If you had a magic wand, what would you change about your family, or its influence at this time in your life? Once you can define a specific goal—such as, "My mother needs to tell me positive—not negative—things about my ability to be a parent"—you can brainstorm about how you might achieve that goal. It is often easier to write letters to family members, telling them what you would like to see change, rather than confronting them in person or by telephone. You may want to write several drafts of your letter, and to have a trusted person review them for you and offer constructive criticism. You may also want to practice what you would say to family members, should they call you or talk to you in person in response to your letter. Rehearse in front of the mirror, keeping focused on your feelings, and using "I" rather than "you" in your sentences.

Families can be powerful influences in our lives; and it can be very difficult to sort these things out on your own. If confronting your family seems overwhelming, you may want to get the added support of professional counseling. An impartial third party may be better equipped than someone close to you to help you decide what changes you want to see. Many therapists are well-schooled in techniques to help you change the role you play in your family of origin. If you're worried about hurting family members by bringing up the issues involved, think about your problem from the perspective of a parent. If you were doing something that was hurting your son or daughter, wouldn't you want your child to tell you, so that you could make the situation better?

If your parents are dead or otherwise unavailable, it's still important to work these issues out of your system. Write letters even if you can't mail them. Putting your thoughts down on paper can do wonders to clarify your feelings. The best insurance against repeating dysfunctional family patterns is to be as conscious and clear about them as possible.

Uninvolved or absent partner.   In many marriages, one partner may in effect be absent because of work demands, travel schedules, or busy lives in general. Perhaps you pictured parenting as a joint venture, but now feel as if you're flying solo. Some new mothers feel this way because of the physical demands of breastfeeding. Mothers, much more often than fathers, take extended leave for infant care. Even though times are changing, many new parents even now have to struggle consciously not to fall into the traditional roles of father as breadwinner and mother as homemaker. We've noticed a tendency in many new fathers to actually increase their time at work postpartum. This appears to be a common way for men to cope with the new responsibilities of being a parent (or adding a child to their family). In the words of one new father, "Suddenly I was responsible for another human being. I felt an overwhelming urge to make more money, work harder, save more to give my baby the best." Work may also provide an arena in which the new father feels in control, compared to the many unknowns of infant care at home. He may spend more time at work because it's at least familiar, and therefore more comfortable. For these many reasons, you may find yourself shouldering what seems like the total burden of infant care and running the household. There are techniques you can use to involve your partner more, with both you and the baby.

You may want to begin by setting up a weekly "date." That can be time out of the house for you and your partner together, dinner together after the baby is in bed, or simply a designated "talk time" to keep in touch with each other's lives. Your relationship is the foundation of your new family, and you will now need to devote time to nurturing it, just as you need to nurture your baby. You need to *plan* time together; otherwise, it can easily get swallowed up by other tasks and activities that seem much more pressing. Sitting together and just listening to music, or cuddling, or taking turns massaging each other's shoulders are other important ways to stay close and keep in touch.

Assigning your partner one specific child-care task each day can also increase his involvement with the baby. You'll get a break as well. Have your partner give the baby a bath each evening, or rock the baby to sleep. It's tempting to have your partner tackle the dishes, rather than a child-care task. But your goal is to involve him with the baby, and to build the infant-parent relationship—as well as to give you a break. Some new fathers may feel uncomfortable about their lack of experience with babies, and may balk at taking on such a task; but, with time, they can develop confidence and may come to treasure their special time with their baby. You may have to "disappear" during this time. Go into your room and close the door, take a shower, go for a walk, or run an errand. Otherwise, you may be tempted to hover, offering comments on how to do the task the "right" way. Your way is not necessarily the only way; your partner may feel comfortable with a different style. Experts say that babies benefit from the different approaches a mother and father bring to childcare. When you remain in the background "directing" the parent-child interaction, you may aggravate your partner's lack of self-confidence, and actually discourage further involvement.

All parents must find their own way to meet their baby's needs. If you correct your partner too much, you may find the whole load of responsibility back in your lap.

In addition to having your partner take charge of one specific child-care task each day, you may want to schedule a morning or evening "off duty" for yourself each week. Your partner can take over then, giving you time for yourself. This is important even for parents who are working full-time. You may feel as if you're already gone too much. But you need to remember that you're a person first, and a parent second: you still need time to devote to nonparental interests.

If setting up structured plans doesn't relieve negative feelings about your partner's absences or lack of emotional involvement, you may want to consult a competent couples therapist.

If your child's father doesn't live with you, please read Chapter 5, which addresses the special needs of single parents.

Loss. There are certain losses that are part of being a new parent. You may feel a real loss of freedom—from being able to come and go as you please, to always having to plan for the baby before you go *anywhere*. You may feel sad about losing your carefree, childless lifestyle. Sleeping until noon on the weekends, staying up late, dancing until dawn may be things of the past. Many women feel that they have lost their "self" and turned into a parent, a person who is foreign to them. "I'm no longer the old me," is a frequent complaint. You may feel sad about losing the specialness of pregnancy. You are no longer the focus of attention and doting; people now smile at the baby, not you. You may feel the loss of the close relationship you had with your physician or midwife. You visit extensively with that person for nine months, trust in them, rely on them, feel cared for by them. Then suddenly that person is "discharging" you, and you will see them only rarely.

You need to allow yourself to acknowledge any of these losses that you feel keenly. They are real. Give yourself permission and time to grieve your losses. Acknowledge the sadness, cry, keep a journal to record your feelings. You need to seek the support of your family in this process as well. You may need to hear from your partner that the loss is real, a confirmation of your need to grieve it, so that you can start to feel better. Don't be afraid to ask for this acknowledgement and support from the people who matter to you.

A death in the family, illness, disability of any close relative, friend, or the baby can significantly affect your feelings postpartum. Other losses, such as moving to another state or town, job changes, or friends moving away can also feel devastating at this time. You may feel as if you should just "cheer up" and forget the loss, focus on the baby instead. You're even likely to hear such things from well-meaning family or friends.

But you need to allow yourself to feel your feelings rather than push them away. Give yourself permission to grieve. Cry, set aside time to feel sad, record your feelings in a journal or letters to loved ones. This is a real loss you have experienced, and you need to grieve it just as you would at any other time in your life. Just because you have a new baby doesn't mean that your feelings of grief are any different or any less powerful. It only means that the grief may be harder to face, and you have less time to take care of your emotional needs. It's still essential that you find the time. And it's important for those around you to realize that you need to grieve, and for them to offer words of encouragement and support as you air your feelings.

If you find that you cannot grieve your losses on your own, you may be able to participate in a local "grief group." Often sponsored by religious or mental health organizations, these groups work as classes, educating participants about the grief process. Having a specific time and place set aside to grieve, as in a group like this, can make working through the grief an easier task. Professional counseling is another option for working through your feelings of loss.

Guilt.   The adjustment of new parents is often complicated by guilt. It's a difficult task to try to maintain your pre-baby life and do a good enough job of meeting your baby's needs as well. You may feel as if you never have enough time for everything you want to do. If you neglect your own needs or your partner or your job, you feel guilty. And you feel guilty if you put any of those priorities above the baby's needs. Guilt just comes with the territory at times. It's normal to want to be at home with the baby if you're at work, and to want a break from the baby if you're at home. Getting yourself on a schedule, so that time is allotted for everyone's needs (including your own), can help. Play with the baby, then do one household task, then take a brief rest break for yourself followed by cuddle time for your partner. Of course, your schedule will be determined by how cooperative or sleepy your baby is, or else on the strength and presence of your support network. You can tell yourself that you are doing it all, just not all at once.

What you say to yourself is equally important in combating "mother guilt." Focus on what you have accomplished rather than what you had to leave undone, and state your accomplishments out loud to yourself. "I got the beds made." "I snuggled with the baby." "I'm doing a good enough job with the housework." "I completed that project on time." Specific accomplishments listed on a piece of paper on your desk or the fridge can remind you that you are making progress. You also may need to allow yourself lower standards and less ambitious goals for a while.

To deal with guilt, social support is again critical. If you are at home, find other at-home parents to meet with on a regular basis. And if you're working out of the home, join a professional women's organization and find some other working mothers to compare notes with.

Some women experience obsessive thoughts about harm that could come to the baby or other loved ones. You may find yourself thinking about throwing the baby down the stairs, or hurting the baby with knives, or simply wishing that the baby would "go away." Along with these thoughts, which most women who experience them feel unable to control, often comes extreme guilt. "What is the matter with me for having such thoughts?" you may ask yourself in horror. And yet these thoughts are quite common, resulting from the biochemical changes in your body (see the section in Chapter 2 on obsessive-compulsive thoughts). You may wish to find someone to talk to who has experienced similar obsessive thoughts. You may be able to find a postpartum support group, or a telephone volunteer (through D.A.D. or P.S.I.—see the Resources section in the back of the book) who can reassure you. You are not a bad person— you're just suffering from changes in your body's chemical balance. It may help to know that women who have such thoughts rarely act on them. You also need to tell yourself that having these thoughts does not mean that you intend to act on them.

It's important to make sure that you have obsessive-compulsive disorder rather than psychosis. Chapter 2 makes these distinctions clear. If you, or anyone around you, have doubts, please consult with a medical professional who is knowledgeable about these disorders.

Often, women who have obsessive thoughts are keenly aware of the importance of their new role as a parent. You may be particularly sensitive to how fragile life is, and how vulnerable your child is. Having these obsessive thoughts may be one way that your body keeps you attuned to that vulnerability, so that you will remain vigilant about your child's safety. However, this can get out of control, so that you focus too much on the dangers your child faces in this world, rather than on the control you do have. Talk to a knowledgeable professional if you feel you cannot see anything but danger for your child ahead.

Body image.   Your body doesn't feel like yours anymore. You may look in the mirror and wonder who it is you're seeing. What happened to your pre-baby body? Just getting dressed in the morning can trigger all kinds of negative feelings about your current shape and weight. Exercise and proper diet are critical to feeling better, of course. Shop smart, stocking up on low-fat, high energy foods like whole-grain breads, nonfat yogurt, fruit, and vegetables. Plan special low-fat snacks for your break times, and make a point of using a special mug or napkin, or setting a flower in a vase at your place. Take a postpartum exercise class where babies are welcome. Get back to an activity you enjoyed pre-baby, such as tennis, golf, or running.

Exercise and diet are important, but so is what you say to yourself. Stating to yourself, or posting on your fridge, "My body is looking better and better every day," or "I can eat just what I need," can give you the feeling that you can control this part of your life. Look in the mirror, and find one feature that you like in your appearance. Then celebrate it some way. Wear a shirt that matches your eyes, or buy a new clip for your hair. The next week, search for another feature you can feel good about right now. Set small goals, and focus on telling yourself you are doing well enough. Your body has changed, and may never be exactly the same as it was before. You may need to grieve this as a significant loss (see the entry on *loss* earlier). Change what you can, and talk yourself into acceptance of what won't change. Your baby loves your body just the way it is.

Try to be loving toward yourself as well. If none of your clothes fit you, buy some attractive clothes that fit your body just as it is now. Don't put off looking your best until you have your old body back, or lose a certain amount of weight. Celebrate your body as it is in the here and now. It's performed miraculous feats and deserves some positive recognition.

Financial stress.   Changing income levels and rising expenses cause financial stress for many new parents. If you and your husband make an effort not to spend more than you take in, the financial strain of having a baby will probably diminish over time. If your financial problems seem overwhelming, you may want to look for the Consumer Credit Counseling Service in your area. This is a nonprofit community agency that can offer advice on budgeting and consolidation of debt.

Attachment.   You may worry about the effects of your postpartum adjustment symptoms on the relationship you are developing with your baby. Attachment or bonding with your baby occurs over the course of time, and is influenced by many factors. Your mood is just one of those factors. While you want to do all you can to take care of yourself and improve your mood, you need to remember that how you feel is not the only influence. Your baby's temperament, the involvement of other adults in your baby's life, and the interaction you and the baby have on your good days all affect the bonding process. And the passage of time will help you build the relationship with your baby, as you begin to feel better. There is no "critical period" for human infants when you either have to "bond" or all is lost. If you miss the first few weeks because of severe symptoms, you can work at the mother-infant relationship when you feel better.

You may feel simple concern about your relationship with the baby, or you may feel that your baby is rejecting you or doesn't like you. Planning time to play with your baby, or simply watch what your baby can do at different stages, is helpful. Borrow or buy a book on what babies can do, such as *Infants and Mothers* by T. Berry Brazelton, or *The New Beyond Peek-a-boo and Pat-a-cake* by Evelyn Munger and Susan Bowdon. Child development and child-care books can give you ideas on how to approach your baby. You may need reassurance that your baby sees you as someone special. Ask your partner or the baby's pediatrician to help you identify the positive ways in which the baby responds to you, if you are unable to identify these on your own. Or have someone videotape an interaction between you and the baby, then watch it at a quiet time. This will allow you to see the baby's responses a bit more objectively—

and will also allow you to gauge your own responses and body language. It takes awhile for babies to begin responding differently to different people, especially if you're bottle-feeding. Be patient; give it time.

Mental health professionals offer parent-child therapy to improve your attachment if you continue to be worried about it later. The family in which you grew up may be influencing your ability to bond with your baby. Working out those family issues in therapy can lead the way to a better relationship with your child.

Relationship difficulties.   One of the major stresses and adjustments in the postpartum period is maintaining the balance in your relationship with your partner. Babies require you to rethink how you have set up your relationship: who takes care of whom, who pays the bills, who makes the money, who has veto power. All the discussions you may have had, and all your expectations and fantasies, often go out the window when you bring the new baby home. The most powerful model in the back of your mind for how a family should be is how your family was when you were growing up. You may be overwhelmed to find yourself in your parents' marriage all of a sudden, acting just as they did and expecting your partner to do the same.

Rather than feeling devastated by these changes in your relationship, be assured that they are completely normal. All couples go through an adjustment period after the birth of a baby. You and your partner need to take it slowly, and realize that you can get back to your previous status if you just don't panic. All the changes that have occurred do not mean that your pre-baby ways of relating are gone for good. They're just lost in the fog for a while. Spend lots of time discussing what you want, how you're feeling, and how you'd like your relationship to be. Stick to wording using "I," not "you." Use concrete examples of behavior you'd like to see. For example, "I like it when you hug me when you come home," is much more positive than, "You never pay attention to me anymore." Remember that you're in this together, and solutions will only come if you work together.

If you and your partner have a stormy relationship history, your previous problems will likely be magnified after your baby arrives. For instance, feeling that your partner is always critical will likely mushroom into a major issue if you are the least bit insecure about parenting. Expect to have to face these ongoing issues as a couple. Counseling is advisable if you are unable to iron out these differences on your own. Do take your conflicts seriously, and seek outside help if you need it; divorce is not uncommon after the birth of a baby. Use all the stresses and strains of the adjustment period as an excuse to rework your relationship into a stronger and more positive bond.

Self-esteem, self-doubt, and identity.   You may find yourself mourning the loss of your "old self" now that you are "just somebody's mother." Questioning who you are or your value as a person is a common concern after the birth of a baby. You may have had a strong identity as a working person, and felt good in that role. But now you may place less emphasis on that part of yourself, or have given it up (for a while or forever) in order to devote more of your energy to parenting. You may feel lost without the old you. Many new mothers feel less valuable without outside income and periodic performance reviews. And caring for an infant does little to bolster self-esteem with the long hours, tiring physical labor, and lack of feedback involved. Your baby never looks up and says, "Good job, mom!" It's no wonder you may question the whole process, and your importance as a part of it. Our society does not put a high premium on parenting. Evidence of this is found everywhere, from the low pay for teachers and child-care workers, to the lack of available training for parents, to the snub you may have experienced at a social gathering when you say that you are "just a mother."

You need a bumper sticker that says, "Motherhood is a proud profession." Raising children to adulthood is an immensely valuable occupation, whether you are home all day or balancing paid work with full-time parenting. You need to recognize your strengths, as a parent and otherwise.

List your strengths on paper and review them every day. List your accomplishments, too, in parenting and in other arenas. If you feel that you have given up everything to devote yourself to your baby, identify a part of your pre-baby self that you would like to revive. Then do it. Have your partner care for the baby so you can take a class, indulge a hobby, develop or improve a skill. Don't be afraid to ask for recognition or a pat on the back from those around you, whether family, friends, or work associates. Most important is how you talk to yourself, however, and value your own achievements, at home and elsewhere. Tell yourself you did a good enough job, that you are doing the best you can do. If you are proud of yourself, and speak up about it, or even show this in your body language, others will take note and respect you, too. If you have serious doubts about your ability in a certain area, take the plunge to improve yourself. Take a class, do some reading, or just experiment with a new way of doing things. Don't be afraid to make mistakes; you can survive a mistake or two. People who doubt themselves improve fastest when they jump right in and attempt to solve the problem, rather than brooding about it for a long time. Even if they don't solve their problem perfectly the first time, they feel better and stronger for having tackled it.

If you feel insecure about your identity, try to picture yourself as a pie chart. Your specialness lies in your different roles or components: you may be a daughter, mother, wife, teacher, tennis player, dancer, cook. Each piece of the pie is important to making you you. When you have a new baby, the mother part may seem to make up most of the pie. Those other pieces are still there, even if they've shrunk to thin wedges. You need to allow yourself time, and find the energy, to develop those other parts of the pie and feel like yourself again. Being your "whole self" is another important way in which taking care of yourself will allow you to nurture your baby.

Getting in Gear

There are many symptoms and issues that may be affecting you throughout the postpartum period, but you can tackle them. Women and their families do get through these difficult times. Set up your plan; persist toward your goal of feeling better. Take care of yourself one step at a time.

You need not be in this battle all alone. Support groups and telephone contact persons are out there, even if they may seem difficult to find at first. You can begin your search with either of the national self-help groups, Depression After Delivery or Postpartum Support International (the telephone numbers are in the Resources Section at the back of this book). Call your local hospital, mental health association, parenting association, or religious organization. Talk to your health-care provider or childbirth educator. If you cannot locate a support group targeted specifically at postpartum adjustment problems, you may be able to find a helpful group that calls itself by another name. Local groups of new mothers may be meeting as breastfeeding support groups, postpartum exercise groups, parenting classes, parent-infant interaction classes or groups, parent-tot play groups, early childhood study groups, or religious groups.

If you do not find a group that's linked to the word "postpartum," look for any group involving new parents. Even if the focus is not on postpartum adjustment problems, there may be much valuable "new parent" support available for you anyway. If all else fails, ask everyone you know for names of other new mothers who might like to meet and share ideas and solutions. Then contact one or more of them, and make an effort to get together on a regular basis. Even a more broadly focused group will immediately reveal that most new parents find the job of parenting tiring, demanding, and confusing. When you see that others struggle to feel good about this life transition, you are less likely to feel that something is wrong with you for feeling dissatisfied. Reading other women's accounts of parenting can ease your adjustment and make you feel less isolated. Our favorite books of this type are included in the Resources Section.

If you still feel overwhelmed after concerted effort on your part, or if the suggestions here do not give you the relief you seek, consult a professional therapist. Use these guidelines as criteria for when to seek professional help:

- When talking out feelings with family, friends, or a support group does not resolve them

- When continuing symptoms of depression are present (for instance, sleeping problems, lack of appetite, severe constipation, not getting dressed all day)

- When you have thoughts about harming yourself or the baby

- When anxiety about everyday problems overwhelms you

See Chapter 7 for ways to find competent help.

5

Unique Needs—Help for Single Mothers, Older Mothers, Adoptive Mothers, and Families with Infertility Issues

The Short Version
(If You're Pressed for Time)

Not every new mother today fits the traditional model for a family containing a husband, a wife, and a baby. If you are one of the many mothers who is older, or single, or who struggled to get pregnant, or adopted a baby, the stress level in your life may be very high. This chapter offers support and ideas to help you face the unique challenges of your untraditional situation.

For new mothers in these categories, **expectations** may contribute greatly to how you feel now. Perhaps you worked toward this goal of having a baby for a long time. You may have expected that achieving your goal would make everything in your life perfect. Or, if you are a single mother who chose to have a baby on her own, you may feel that you worked against tough odds to have this baby—but now that you have it, you expect everything to go smoothly. If your expectations postpartum are that the worst is now over, or that you should be completely happy to finally have this baby in your arms, you may be sorely disappointed. Having a new baby is difficult, tiring, and overwhelming at times. If you expect it to be otherwise—or if you expect to have all the answers because you're older, more experienced, wanted it so badly, and so on—you may find yourself feeling like a failure, because things just aren't that way. You need to identify your expectations about motherhood, and the myths or beliefs that underlie them, and then sort out the unrealistic expectations from the more reasonable ones.

This job of being a new parent will not be any different because of the way you got here. New babies don't know what their parents have been through up to this point. They still cry, need to eat and dirty their diapers a lot, and ignore your ideas about schedules and organization. You need to throw those ideas out as well, and take things one day at a time, instead of feeling frustrated because things aren't going according to the grand plan you have in your head about what things *should* be like.

Another issue that mothers in these categories share is a **feeling of being all alone**. You may not know another new parent who is older, single, adoptive, and so on. You may feel the lack of models for how to take on this job. Because new mothers like yourself may be harder to find than the "typical" new mother in her twenties, with a husband in tow, you may need to work harder to find a supportive group of people in the same boat. But making friends and developing a support network of even one or two people is even more critical for you, because you don't fit the usual model. You may have to work hard to find soul mates, but the effort will pay off.

The third issue shared by this category of mothers is **physical stress and fatigue**. Older mothers may find themselves more tired because of their age. Single mothers may suffer more because they may have no one to give them relief from baby tasks. And women who have had infertility troubles may be more at risk biochemically for physical symptoms. Whatever hormonal problems contributed to your infertility may still be operating, making you more at risk for physical and emotional strain. Adoptive mothers may think they don't have to worry about fatigue, because they bypassed the physical stress of pregnancy and birth. But they still need to take care of the baby all day and night, which is a strain in itself. What this means for you is that you need to take extra care of yourself. You need to rest more, nap more, exercise, and eat right, just like any other new mother. You can't expect to just keep going nonstop. No one can. Take care of yourself physically, and arrange to take breaks. These measures are critical for all new mothers.

Older Mothers—Issues and Answers

Lifestyle changes.   You may feel as if your life has gone from control to chaos. It likely has. To work on tolerating the changes involved, you can

- Focus on the positive aspects of your situation. What do you love about it?

- Find one area of your life where you have control, and focus on this. Recite to yourself, "I am in control of neatness in this one room," or "I can work on getting my body back by exercising," or "I can still feel in charge at work."

Aging parents.   You may be what is called the "sandwich generation," caring for aging parents as well as young children. Find some other people who are doing what you're doing, and talk with them. Structuring your time, and delegating work to others (family members, health-care workers) when you can will also help you handle the load. Don't forget time off for yourself. You can't nurture others if your pitcher is empty.

Women with Infertility Issues or Women Who Have Adopted

Guilt and worth as a woman.   You may feel like a failure "as a woman" if you had difficulty having a baby in the "natural" way. You need to congratulate yourself for having the strength and determination to bring this baby into your life. Make a list of things you do well as a parent, rather than dwelling on how you got to this point. Try not to play "what if," which is common with adoptive parents: "What if she were my biological daughter? Would I understand her cries better?" Thoughts like this only make you unsure of yourself. Support from other mothers in the same situation is critical now.

Single Mothers

Feeling loved and meeting your needs.   Even though you have your baby now, you still have adult needs—for companionship, for love, for feeling important. Work to get those needs met from adult sources. Your baby can make you feel loved at times, but it's important not to rely on a child for feeling good about yourself. First of all, children can't be relied on to let you know you're doing a good job. Secondly, you need to work on meeting the baby's needs, not on the baby meeting yours. Finding ways to feel good about yourself among adults is an important consideration to squeeze into your day.

Mourning your loss of the ideal.   You may feel sad because you are not sharing this life stage with a partner, as you probably imagined you would all your life. You may have lots of anger about this. Allow yourself time to cry, to be angry and get those feelings out in a safe way, away from the baby. Write, pound a pillow, scream in the shower. Those feelings are real, and you need to take care of them.

Although some women facing these special challenges may have a hard road ahead, they rise to these challenges every day. You need to work at taking care of yourself physically and emotionally, at having fun, and getting breaks or help from others. You need to plan your days quite rigorously to include everything important to your care and the baby's. You need to find others who are in the same boat. And you need to pat yourself on the back and recognize all the good things you're doing well.

Exercise
Two Minutes for Yourself

Take a kitchen timer with you into the bathroom. Set it for two minutes, then step into the shower. Turn on the water, fast and furiously. As you let the water flow over you, shout out your anger. "I am so mad! I am furious that I feel so rotten!" Keep raging for two full minutes. Let the water wash that anger off you and down the drain. Imagine your words and feelings swirling away with the water.

After the timer rings, finish your shower, but imagine that there's healing balm in the water. Every place it touches you, it makes you feel stronger, healthier, and more relaxed.

5

Unique Needs—Help for Single Mothers, Older Mothers, Adoptive Mothers, and Families with Infertility Issues

In our society today, there no longer seems to be one "right" way to have a baby. For your parents' generation, the common pattern was to be married one or two years, and then to start a family. Since most people married in their late teens or early twenties, that placed most new parents in their early twenties. Current statistics tell us that more and more older women are having babies, and a significant percentage of those women are single parents. According to the *Statistical Handbook on Women in America*, since 1975 birth rates have been rising only in women between the ages of 30 to 44. For younger groups of women, birth rates are declining or holding steady. In other words, more and more women are delaying childbirth until they are in their thirties or beyond. U.S. Census data indicate that the percentage of children born to unmarried women rose from 10.7 percent of all births in 1970 to 25.7 percent in 1988. Because not every new mother is living out the "two-parents-in-their-twenties" model, this chapter will address some of the unique stresses and needs that are part of the territory of alternative lifestyle choices.

Older Mothers

Just how old do you have to be to be considered an older mother? Most women are reluctant to label themselves as "older," and with good reason—the word is burdened with a truckload of negative associations in our culture. But, for some reason, the medical community applies the label without mercy: pregnant women over 30 have "geriatric mother" written in their chart in many hospitals across the country! No matter how old you are, this section may be helpful to you if you feel out of step with your peers in terms of childbearing. If most of your friends, relatives, and coworkers have children who are much older than yours, you may find reassurance and helpful suggestions in this chapter.

"Older mothers" used to be popularly defined as anyone over 30; then the age limit stretched to over 35, and now, in some parts of the country, may not be applied until a woman is past 40. As more and more women choose to begin bearing children later in life, the label "older mother" is more sparingly applied. Perhaps it will soon be reserved for those post-menopausal women choosing to carry a child by the grace of modern science and lots of ready cash.

What is important in the equation is how *you* define yourself, and how you manage your postpartum adjustment. In *Sooner or Later: The Timing of Parenthood in Adult Lives*, Pamela Daniels and Kathy Weingarten describe three reactions to "mid-life" parenting. In the first, a new baby is seen as a "supplemental experience." The parents easily work the baby into their existing lifestyle. They do not change much, and roll along as if nothing has happened. The second style is the "new chapter" approach. There may be an abrupt shift in priorities and the way in which the parent structures life day to day. These parents may stay home more, become more safety conscious, change their diet and exercise routines, and save money after spending freely for years. In the third style—"the crunch"— new parents find the reality of having a baby difficult to accept. They feel unable to be a good parent or do anything right, whereas before everything in their lives was on an even keel. Their balance is all upset, and the experience feels completely traumatic. This sense of a "crunch" is often aggravated by unrealistic expectations about parenthood, or by a baby with health or temperamental problems.

Issues for Older Mothers

Expectations.   The primary hurdle for many new mothers of whatever age is their expectations. Prospective parents can spin beautiful dreams about being a mom or a dad. It can be quite upsetting when the reality of parenthood doesn't even vaguely resemble that pretty picture in your head. Older mothers may have the greatest expectations of all. They can easily fall prey to the idea that their greater age and experience will give them an edge in this parenting business. You, or others around you, may feel that you will *know* better how to be a parent, because you have such a wealth of experience on which to draw. You may have even more invested in the notion of being "perfect" because you delayed childbearing for such a long time. As Carol Dix writes in *The New Mother Syndrome*, you may feel you have to do everything right because society expects mothers to be younger, and so you need to prove yourself. You may be extremely used to having most things in life go your way. You've probably worked hard to mold your destiny, and make it the way you planned, right down to the timing of parenthood. And you may, quite logically, expect things to continue in this vein.

These sorts of expectations can cause immense confusion and frustration as you discover how impossible they are in reality. You can't control what kind of pregnancy or birth experience you have; you can't order a child made up to your specifications. What sort of flip-flops your hormones are going to do postpartum is a big unknown. Having years of experience in the work world may give you an edge in handling a new baby, or it may not. The day-to-day tediousness of caring for an infant may come as a shock to you. You may have put motherhood off, waiting until you were really sure, only to discover that all your earlier doubts came back when reality set in. For most people, taking care of an infant just isn't all that much fun, especially when you're on duty 24 hours a day. You have little or no control over when your baby eats, sleeps, cries, or needs changing. Suddenly you are working on someone else's timetable, after being in charge of your own timetable for years. No matter how organized you are, or how much time you allow, the baby is just bound to poop or spit up all over both of you just as you've gotten him all dressed up and you're ready to go out the door.

You may be asking yourself, "Did I wait too long to have a child?" On bad days, you may wonder if you made the wrong decision to have a baby at all. Of course you feel badly: nothing has gone according to plan—so much for your glorious expectations!

Even though these concerns may be slightly amplified if you're older, they are still common among all new parents of whatever age. We've tried to address some of the special concerns of older new mothers below.

Physical stress and fatigue.   Because you're not 22 years old anymore you may experience greater physical stress and fatigue during pregnancy and the postpartum period. Many mothers note this difference between the way they felt with the first child and the way they feel with the second or third, even if the children are only two or three years apart. It may or may not be reassuring to note that you feel more tired, more worn out by the physical demands of childbearing, just because your body is older.

However, a lack of physical stamina is not the only contributor to your overwhelming sense of exhaustion. As an older mother, your sense of loss of your old self may be even stronger than it would be for a younger woman. You may have had more of an old self to lose—you were probably more sure of yourself overall than you were a decade ago. This makes for a greater contrast between the old self-confident you and the new you, who is a mother now, facing all sorts of uncertainties. This sudden decrease in your self-confidence can contribute to a sense of being overwhelmed and fatigued.

Disappointed expectations can play a role in your fatigue as well. Because you want everything with this new baby to be just right, you may be denying your negative feelings more urgently. You try to ignore your impatience, fatigue, and frustration with this new situation. As a result, you may be pushing yourself too hard, not taking breaks or rests, or ignoring your body's signals of fatigue. This can lead to even greater exhaustion and even collapse, because you are not taking care of yourself as you need to at this demanding time.

Lack of role models.   Social isolation may be the worst for older mothers. You may be the only person you know who has an infant. Your friends and contemporaries may have teenagers, or at least school-age children. It may be very difficult to find other new mothers your age, and you may be without a social support network as a result. Feeling so alone can worsen your doubt about what you've done to your life by having a baby. Not having another new mother with whom you can compare symptoms, pointers, and problems can leave you feeling very lost. New parenting is always made easier by having a crew of friends who are fighting the same battles.

Aging parents.   If you're older than the average new mother, chances are that your parents (or your spouse's parents) are also older than the average new grandparents. This can create problems in two ways. First of all, if the grandparents are older, they may be less able to provide the physical caretaking that is so helpful in the postpartum period. Your mother and/or mother-in-law may be unable to come and help with the housework, the baby, and your recovery if they are in their seventies rather than in their fifties. They may not be strong enough or patient enough for babysitting or the other tasks that grandparents have traditionally provided in families. The situation will be even more complicated if grandparents are in ill health. You and your partner may find yourselves in the role of caretaker for two generations: your new baby and your aging parents. This can add great stress to the already tough job of adjusting to parenthood.

Lifestyle changes, from control to chaos.   In *The New Mother Syndrome*, Carol Dix explains that the older mother may be used to a certain amount of control, competence, and independence in her life. You may look at freedom, privacy, and tranquility as inalienable rights—and yet they vanish with a new baby. Babies create an environment in which messiness, chaos, and crisis are the norm. Baby equipment, baby schedules, and baby's needs all wreak havoc on your controlled, calm life. This is reality, and the reality goes on for years as babies turn into toddlers and then teenagers. Children have minds of their own, and it is often necessary to compromise your own needs to meet theirs. This can be a very difficult adjustment.

Carer and financial changes.   You may not be making any changes in your career plans or financial status. But it's common for older mothers to make big changes in this regard. After all, you may have waited this long to have children so you'd have enough financial security to be able to take an extended leave and stay home with your baby. You may find yourself surprised at any resentment you feel about career changes or financial sacrifices, when you chose them willingly. Just because you made those choices doesn't mean that the adjustment will be easy. You may find the loss of professional identity painful—imagine how your partner would feel if he suddenly found himself without a career! You may not like your financial dependence on your spouse, after many years of independence. All of these feelings are real and legitimate, even though they may take you by surprise.

Self-Care for Older Mothers

Feeling good in the postpartum period begins with your self-care plan, no matter what your age. Make sure you've read Chapter 4, which covers the basics. Special considerations for older mothers are covered below.

Scale down your expectations.   Disappointed expectations may be responsible for the lion's share of your negative feelings. You may have set yourself up by expecting too much, too soon. Perhaps you've bought into the idea that because you are older and more experienced, you'll always make smart choices and do a terrific job as a parent. Perhaps you fully expected to step into the role of Supermom, able to breastfeed your baby while negotiating mergers, all prepared to host a dinner for eight that evening (after arranging the flowers, doing 180 sit-ups, and cleaning out the garage).

It's time to readjust those expectations, now that you know a little more about the realities of life postpartum. Divide a piece of paper into three columns. Then make a list of the images you had of yourself in your new role. For each image, think about the myth that may be hovering behind it. For instance, if you saw yourself baking bread and making baby clothes while your baby slept, the underlying myth might be something like: "I'm organized, creative, and capable—I should be able to do it all." After you've identified four or five such images and the myths behind them, write a statement in the third column that gets you off the hook. In the example above, you might write, "Sure I'm organized, creative, and capable—but I'm under extraordinary physical and emotional pressures right now. It's perfectly fine if I just manage to take care of myself and the baby, without accomplishing one single thing more!"

Myths and expectations are sneaky. They may be operating in your brain, influencing your behavior and mood, without your knowledge that you're buying into these false ideas. If you're having trouble identifying the expectations you're imposing on yourself, and the myths behind them, you may want to air your ideas with a trusted friend, family member, or counselor.

Write yourself some positive affirmations, as suggested in Chapter 4. These messages can take the form of general reminders—such as, "You can be a good enough parent," or "Every parent makes mistakes—children are enormously resilient"—written on note cards or self-adhesive notes, and posted in obvious places. You may want to put them on your mirror, on your checkbook, on the fridge—anywhere they'll come to your attention on a daily basis.

Do whatever you can to counteract your expectations of perfection. Each morning you may need to get out your three-column list and review it, repeating the third-column statements—those that get you off the hook—out loud. You *can* learn to do this job of parenting, and do it well. But give yourself a break and avoid scolding yourself for not living up to some totally unrealistic ideal.

Everyone makes mistakes, gets exhausted, has bad days and negative feelings, and struggles to feel good as a parent. You're not exempt from the struggle just because you have a certain number of candles on your birthday cake. There's nothing wrong with you for feeling rotten or disappointed or both. Own up to realities, then take steps to remedy the situation.

Focus on the positive.   Aside from the myths, there really are advantages to being older in this parenting business. You may, in fact, be more mature and better prepared emotionally to focus on someone else's needs. Your priorities in life may be clearer than a younger person's. Your value system has been well thought out, and you've had time to test it over the years. You have more perspective. You may have a secure idea of who you are, and a clear sense that you are capable of competence. Of course, you may lose track of your self-confidence in the war zone of life with a new baby.

To give yourself a boost, take a deep breath and close your eyes. Tell yourself that the competence and self-assurance that you had in other arenas can transfer to your motherhood role. You are learning a new job. As with all new jobs, there's an apprenticeship period during which you're learning lots all at once. But you have a good foundation to build on.

Now take another deep breath, and tell yourself that it's okay if it takes you a long time to adapt, and it's okay when you make mistakes—because you will make mistakes. Everyone does—even older moms.

You may be more financially secure than you were ten years ago. This may mean that you'll have fewer money worries than you would have had then. Perhaps you're able to pay for some of the help that can make such a difference during this transition time, such as babysitters, housecleaning help, and meal delivery. Take advantage of all the hard work you've done in previous years by letting yourself reap the benefits of these sources of paid support, if at all possible.

Another advantage of your age may be that you are more health-conscious than a younger mother would be. You may have a more real-istic sense of the physical strains and risk to your body that come with not taking care of yourself. You've lived in your body longer, know how it works, and may have learned the importance of good maintenance dur-ing stressed times. This is one of those times. Emphasize those good self-care habits you have developed through your adult life. Good diet, exercise, and rest still go a long way toward promoting your physical and mental health, even if you feel like a wreck now, and your body seems at the mercy of fluctuating hormones. Be happy that you have enough sense and enough practice to take good care of yourself.

Develop a support network.   If you feel as if you're the only mother ever to embark on this new baby adventure at such an advanced age, you definitely need to find a new parent group containing some other older mothers. This may seem daunting if there's no one who meets the description in your immediate circle of acquaintances. But you can take solace in the statistics. If more and more older women are having babies—and they are—there have to be others like you out there some-where. Start asking around. Talk to your childbirth educator, your min-ister or rabbi, your child's pediatrician or your obstetrician, your local mental health association, parenting centers, or community organizers. Keep your eyes open wherever there are moms and babies, and be pre-pared to seize the opportunity to start up a conversation. Carry cards with you that give your name and telephone number. Always keep a pen handy. talk to every person you know—someone is bound to have a sis-ter-in-law, cousin, neighbor, or friend who's in the same boat. then make an effort to get together with even one other older mother on a regular basis. It's wonderful what two people can give to each other; just the feeling that "you are not alone" can brighten your day. Be ready to make the first move, for that is an important step in the business of self-care.

Remember the couple.   For older parents, who may have lived to-gether as a childless couple for a long time, it can be very painful to make the adjustment from exclusive focus on each other to having almost no time together at all. Making your relationship a continuing priority is of premier importance to creating a happy family. You and your partner need to find ways to remind yourselves that your relationship matters. The easiest way to do this is to schedule "couple time" into your day. Set aside ten minutes at 9 p.m. to ask about each other's day. Arrange for a weekly date, when you get out together without the baby. This need not be elaborate; coffee or a walk in the park can work as well as a din-ner-movie-dancing affair. The important thing is that you are saying to each other, "We are important, too." And you are saying that with actions, not just words.

Women with Infertility Issues

You may have worked for a number of years to finally get to this point, your precious baby in your arms. Many women who have expe-rienced difficulty getting pregnant find a very big gap between what they hoped for and the reality of a new baby. You really wanted a baby, and your behavior for a number of years may have been focused almost ex-clusively on that goal. If you wanted this so badly, why do you feel so rotten now that you have it? The guilt may be great at this time. There must really be something the matter with me, you think. Expectations, once again, may be the culprit.

The particular expectations that go with desperate hope.   After investing so much of your time, emotional energy, and perhaps money in having a baby, it's natural to think that achieving your goal will solve all your problems and make you happy. You finally have what you want. But you still don't feel good. That may be because you pictured bringing up a baby as an easy and joyful process. You knew labor would be dif-ficult—you had lots of training to prepare you. The hard part should be over now, and the fun beginning!

Maybe you're bumping up nose to nose against the reality that new babies are demanding, exhausting, and time-consuming little critters. The process of caring for and adjusting to a new baby is wearing for anyone. This will be true for you even though you've tried so hard and worked so much to have a baby. You need to recognize that reality. Even with your heart's desire in your arms and the fulfillment of all your dreams, your life still isn't going to be perfect.

Many women who've gone through the agony of trying for years to get pregnant may have lost perspective about other trials in their lives. You may have thought that achieving this goal would make any other problems seem unimportant. Certainly the stress of infertility treatment and deciding whether to adopt can influence a couple's relationship. And some of that stress may be relieved by finally reaching the goal of having a baby. But it's equally likely that you'll trade the stresses of longing for a baby for the normal stress of adjusting to parenthood together. If you had marital conflict before your fertility struggle was rewarded, that conflict isn't going to just go away. The old myth about babies "fixing marriages" is just not true. You'll still have issues in your marriage to work out, if those issues existed before your baby was born.

After pouring so much of your hope and energy into getting pregnant, you may feel a little at sea after your baby arrives. Hope can be a kind of occupation in itself—after your hope has been fulfilled, that part of you that stayed focused on hoping may feel rather unemployed. It's like people who wish and hope for money, and then suddenly win the lottery—they probably feel great for a while, but then it dawns on them that they're still stuck with being who they are, complete with all their old fears, regrets, insecurities, and limitations. Having your fondest dream fulfilled won't transform you into someone else—you'll simply be who you were, only you have a baby now. People don't live "happily ever after" in real life as they do in fairy tales. Life goes on, with all its muddle and complications.

Guilt and worth as a woman.   You may be plagued by guilt about how badly you've felt since the baby arrived. How can you feel so miserable, you ask yourself, when you wanted this baby so intensely? Many women who have experienced infertility problems already have doubts about their basic worth as a woman. Not only did you have a hard time getting pregnant, but now you have negative feelings toward your baby. It's easy to come to the mistaken conclusion that there's something the matter with you as a woman for being anything less than ecstatically happy all the time. "If I were in working order as a woman, I would have been able to get pregnant sooner," you may tell yourself; or "I would love every moment of being a mother if I weren't so deficient." The reality of motherhood as a difficult, demanding, exhausting job can get lost in the crossfire of self-doubt and blame.

Increased biochemical risk.   Research suggests that women who have had difficulty getting pregnant have higher rates of postpartum adjustment problems. This may indicate greater hormonal influence on these women's moods. In other words, if the hormonal balance in your body was out of whack, causing infertility, your hormones may have to struggle for balance postpartum. As you know by now, most postpartum adjustment problems are caused at least in part by the biochemical free-for-all that goes on in a woman's body after she has a baby. What you are going through now is not your fault. Because you had trouble getting pregnant, you have to allow your body extra time to find its balance, and give yourself extra nurturing to weather the process.

Issues related to adoption.   Many parents who adopt are faced with an issue that's peculiar to their situation: little time to prepare emotionally for the arrival of their baby. More and more adoptions are open, with the birth mother even inviting the adoptive parents to pregnancy checkups and into the delivery room. However, many hopeful couples still find that they get a call from the adoption agency at work one day, with the happy news that "tomorrow you can come get this baby." Two days is not adequate time to prepare emotionally. You may not have made physical preparations, such as buying baby gear or setting up a nursery, because you wanted to protect yourself from "getting your hopes up." And so, suddenly, you have too much to do and think about. You are catapulted into the role of parenting, without the usual gradual adjustment process of nine months of pregnancy. This can leave you feeling very unsure of yourself, wondering how in the world you're going to handle it.

A second issue adoptive parents face, which may continue throughout their lives, is the "what if" game. Most adoptive parents question themselves on many levels. "What if the baby were not adopted? Would I still have so many doubts about how to be a parent? Would I still feel so negative, so lost, blue, and exhausted?" You can torment yourself endlessly with this variety of second-guessing. You will always wonder how things might have been if this were your biological child. And this question may be particularly strong if the new experience of parenthood seems less rosy than you had anticipated.

Developing a Self-Care Plan

Bring your expectations into line with reality. Just because you worked for this new baby for many years does not mean that your baby will sleep more, cry less, or be easier to understand than if you had gotten pregnant long ago. You are subject to the same rules as any other new parents. You still cannot do everything perfectly or control anyone but yourself. Taking care of a newborn is still demanding, exhausting, uncertain work. It's perfectly normal to feel tired, grumpy, insecure, and doubtful. You need to make sure your expectations are realistic. Raising this child to adulthood will be a tough job. But you're as well-equipped as any other parent.

There's no connection between length of time trying to conceive and quality of parenting. You can read parenting books, learn, reassure yourself, and keep your eyes set on the goal of being a "good enough" parent. You are just like any other parent, in that the way you will get through this adjustment period is to take care of yourself as best you can. Stay focused on the realities of the situation, and don't blame yourself for the difficulties.

Finding support. Knowing other parents who have suffered through infertility, or who've adopted, can be particularly healing for this time in your life. You may have to work to develop your own network if there's not an existing one in your area. Organizations such as Resolve, Inc., which provide support to people with fertility problems, may be a place to find others like yourself who now have babies. For adoptive parents, adoption agencies may offer groups to take you beyond those first days at home with your baby. Find several parents in similar situations, and then work to meet and talk with them on a regular basis. If the group only meets once a month, meet with individual members for coffee in between. The more you can see how your concerns are shared by others in the same boat, the better you'll be able to maintain your perspective on your own life. This ultimately will help you to let go of some of your feelings of guilt, self-doubt, and second-guessing.

A word to adoptive parents.   You may think that because you did not endure the physical changes of pregnancy and birth, you do not need special care after your baby comes to live with you! You may think that your excitement will carry you through these exhausting first months. Think again. You need to set the same limits on yourself as any biological parent. You need a rest period each day. You need to sleep when the baby sleeps. After all, you are up with the baby at night, too. You need to limit visitors to certain times, and not feel that you must be ready to entertain at any and all hours. You need to let guests serve themselves; do not expect to be the perfect hostess. You also need to ask for (and accept offers of) help from family and friends. Meals, errand running, household chores—all still must be done, and you probably feel just as overwhelmed as any biological mom. You need to reserve your energy for taking care of the baby and yourself, if at all possible, just as if you had delivered this baby yourself. The stress of trying to do it all is just as great for you—so please follow the advice on physical and emotional caretaking outlined in Chapter 4.

Single Mothers

Facing a new baby largely on your own can be an overwhelming task for any woman. It's quite normal for a new mother to feel stressed, fatigued, unsure of herself, and easily moved to tears or anxiety. When she is tackling parenthood without another adult to provide reassurance and respite, the task can seem overwhelming.

All new mothers need nurturing and support. Single mothers may find that they can accomplish all the child-care tasks, but sorely miss a backup system to provide breaks, back rubs, and breadwinning. This lack can be a huge drain on a new mother's energy. Essentially, the need for self-care and social support in the postpartum period is even more important for the single parent, and harder to squeeze into a crowded day. Exhaustion and feelings of isolation are quite common and understandable in the single mother. You are expected to give, give, give all day long to your infant, with no built-in mechanism to get your own needs met. Maggie Comport, in her book *Surviving Motherhood*, describes the single mother's plight as "a bottomless well of giving . . . while she herself is emotionally starving."

Expectations can be a big stumbling block for the single parent as well. This is especially true if you chose to get pregnant and raise this baby on your own, rather than if you're single now because of death, divorce, or an unplanned pregnancy. You likely had the same glowing ideals in your head about the lovely, cuddly times you and this baby would share—snuggled on the bed at the end of a tiring, but fulfilling day—as does any new mother. The reality may seem quite ugly and glaring to you by contrast, now that the hard, exhausting work of newborn care has begun. Resentment and anger can surface as you work to meet the baby's needs with no one there to meet your needs in turn. Be reassured that feeling fatigued, angry, resentful, and overwhelmed is common in all new parents.

In addition to expectations about parenting itself, you may have great expectations about your ability to cope. If you chose this path, you likely believed that you would be able to triumph as a single mother. As Carol Dix suggests in *The New Mother Syndrome*, you may expect the best of yourself, and so deny any emotional problems. Single mothers may have particular trouble admitting that things aren't going well. To do so feels like admitting failure.

If you are here not by choice, but by circumstance, you may not connect your emotional turmoil to the birth and your adjustment to parenting. You may see your unhappiness solely as the result of your situation, which may cause you to ignore the special measures for self-care that all new mothers need to follow "to keep their pitchers full."

Unique Aspects of Single Parenting

Social ostracism.   "In a world which assumes Mama Bear, Papa Bear, and Baby Bear, people who are one bear short often find themselves feeling ostracized," says Cynthia Copeland Lewis in her book, *Mother's First Year*. Although single parenting is increasingly common, you may still feel self-conscious about not fitting the traditional pattern you see everywhere around you. Social acceptance of single mothers may be greater than it was 20 years ago. But the issue is still a hot one as you may recall from the Murphy Brown-Dan Quayle altercation in 1992. Murphy Brown, lead character on the television series of the same name, chose to have her baby as a single parent. Dan Quayle, in his capacity as Vice President of the United States at the time, criticized the program for its lack of "family values." All hell broke loose after that, with a bitter and often comic exchange of criticism from both sides, and an astonishing amount of public interest. As a single mother you'd have to be living on the moon not to be aware of the widespread disapproval that many people in our society feel perfectly comfortable expressing, even as you struggle to parent your baby on your own. Many single parents have resolved this issue in their own lives, but still feel anguish when society scorns or pities them. And they worry tremendously about how their single status will influence their child. Loneliness, guilt, frustration, and fear are all understandable in the single mother trying to make a go of it on her own.

Feeling loved and meeting needs.   You may have hoped that having this baby to love would relieve some of your feelings of aloneness. It may, but infant companionship is a poor substitute for the adult variety everyone needs. Many single mothers find themselves plagued by fierce protectiveness for their infants. In *The New Mother Syndrome*, Carol Dix suggests that single mothers may feel overprotective because of their own feelings of being unloved and alone.

If you're depending exclusively on this baby and your new family life to relieve your loneliness, you might feel extremely fearful about your child's safety. If something were to happen to your child, your feelings of loneliness, rejection, and being unloved would return in full force. Of course, every new mother fears for her child's safety—but as a single parent you have all your eggs in one basket, as it were. The stakes are higher.

Many single mothers find that the myths and expectations they harbor worsen their feelings of being alone and unlovable. Before you were even pregnant, you likely had a picture in your head about what a new family should look like. Confronting the daily reality that you are in this alone may feel like rubbing salt in a wound. You're constantly reminded that this is not what you had envisioned. You may have always imagined having a partner supporting you through this major life event. The fact that you're on your own now may make you feel that you're a complete failure at relationships, or simply unlovable.

At the same time, when your baby responds to you with a smile, a coo, or snuggling into your shoulder, you can feel very loved indeed. It may grow all too easy to transfer your adult needs for love and affirmation into your relationship with your baby. Focusing intensely on your baby is appropriate for a while, and part of the normal bonding process. But it can be especially difficult for a single mother to maintain some balance between her relationships with other adults and her relationship with her child.

It's impossible to love your child too much; but children cannot meet—and should not be asked to meet—their parents' adult needs. Single mothers, like all other parents, must get their adult needs met by other adults.

This is true for your own sake as well. Your children's needs come first while they're very young, and it's fitting for them to be the focus of much of your attention. But children—very quickly, it seems—grow up, and eventually leave home. To forsake all other relationships because you are getting what you need from your child is to create great pain for yourself in the long run.

If you're gone from your child all day while you're at work, it can seem like an insurmountably difficult task to try to get out for a social event of your own in the evening, or even to take time out for exercise. You may not have the resources to pay for babysitting. You may not have someone reliable with whom you can leave the baby while you take a break. Other people may overlook you as a prospective partner or even companion because you have a child. Women friends may assume you have no time, and men may assume you're unavailable by virtue of your status as a parent. It can be extremely difficult to get your needs met in this situation.

Mourning your loss of the ideal.   Single mothers may find themselves plagued by feelings of sadness or anger at having a baby alone. This is not what they ever expected to do. It's common to hope that, when you do have a baby, you'd be in a supportive, committed relationship.

It's important to allow yourself time to grieve the loss of this ideal. You're not in the relationship you always imagined. You miss the attention, physical warmth, and sexual intimacy of a committed relationship. You miss having someone to confide in, to share decisions—to share your pleasure in watching your baby grow and change.

If you're divorced, or separated from the baby's father, or your partner has died, it's critical that you work through your feelings of loss and grief. Whether you're missing a real person, or the loss of your ideal, you still need to distinguish the guilt and anger caused by your situation from your guilt and anger having to do with the baby and all the normal stresses of motherhood. Making this distinction will make it easier to find ways to feel better on both counts.

Lack of role models.   Even though the number of single mothers is rising, you may not personally know someone who has lived successfully through this tough situation. There are few obvious examples of real women who are coping well with being a single mother. Maybe some movie stars do it—but think of the extraordinary resources at their disposal! It's difficult to study and learn from the ins and outs, the day-to-day trivia of success as a single parent, when you have no one to watch who is several steps ahead of you.

A lowered standard of living.   Many single mothers find themselves faced with a drop in their standard of living. You may choose not to work for a while, to devote yourself to your child. You need to adjust to the decrease in your income, whether you're a single mother by choice or through death or divorce. Considerable stress comes from being the sole breadwinner, and being faced with the increase in expenses that a baby brings about. If your finances were tight before, now they may seem even more restrictive.

Self-Care for Single Mothers

Single mothers need to take care of their own needs just as any new mother must. If you are to fill this role all alone, with no one to give you breaks, planning to get your own needs met is of critical importance. You cannot be a "bottomless well of giving" if you are running on empty yourself.

The first step is to give yourself permission to be a human being as well as a parent. You have a self that needs fun, satisfaction, companionship, entertainment, and rest. Learn that you will be a better parent if you nurture the other parts of yourself along with nurturing your child.

Adjust your expectations.   After giving yourself permission to take care of yourself, you may need to tackle some of your expectations about yourself as a parent. Do you think you can be Supermom? Are you sure you can excel at work, parenting, making your home a nice place to be, and still have time for ballroom dancing lessons, the PTA, and the League of Women Voters? Think again. No one can do it all. The important aspect to focus on is being a "good enough" parent. All parents make mistakes, and the majority of children turn out to be responsible, loving human beings. You may need to work on being more realistic and allowing yourself to not do everything perfectly. Leave the toys out on the floor. Fail to make the bed. Put some energy into different priorities, such as rocking your baby or soaking in the tub yourself. You can even scream at your baby, or yourself, now and then. Separate the action from the person. In other words, you can goof up in one area, one evening, and still be a good person. You can make a mistake with your child, and later apologize. Aim for a balance, with mistakes and triumphs adding up to a good enough job. Of course, if you feel the mistakes greatly outweigh the successes, you may want to talk about your situation with a professional therapist—especially if you fear you might harm yourself or your child.

You also should expect to feel negative at times. This is a time-consuming, exhausting job you are undertaking, especially as you're doing it on your own. Expect to have trouble keeping your cool at times. Have a plan in place for taking a quick break, and replenishing yourself with a distracting activity, such as a shower, a walk, a phone call, or even punching a pillow. Expect to have to struggle to get some time for yourself, but expect to take on that struggle anyway. Try not to expect that you will be better at any of this than the next mom. Give yourself credit for being a human being, and expect to learn new habits, efficiency tricks, and ways to meet your own needs. Work to find small ways to make yourself feel good. Try to see reading ten pages a day in a novel as positive, a small step in the right direction, rather than focusing on how many more pages you would like to have read.

Focus on the positive.   While it may be difficult to see the good side of being a single parent when everything is looking bleak, focusing on the positive might be reassuring to you. There are actually some benefits to single parenting. You may have greater control over raising your child the way you think it should be done. You don't have to negotiate every fine detail of parenting philosophy with someone else. You have greater freedom to do things the way *you* want to do them. No one will tell you that you're always dressing the baby too warmly, or that you need to let her do things more on her own. Later on, your child may really enjoy having you to herself on a daily basis. Children are greedy about parental time, and you may avoid conflicts about balancing your attention between your child and your partner.

Another benefit of single parenting is that society in general tends to be much less critical if you leave your child during the day to earn a living. Married mothers must routinely face such criticism. As Carol Dix points out in *The New Mother Syndrome*, you may also get more help from others, because they realize that you have no partner there with you to pitch in. People may view your situation more realistically, while they may romanticize new parenting for married women.

Social support.   As for any new parent, having contact with others in the same boat can be incredibly affirming. Search for a single parent support group, and find a way to attend. If you cannot find a group, talk to everyone you know about their acquaintances who are also parenting alone. Then arrange to get together, let the children play, and share your experiences. You may find a mentor this way, or at least a sympathetic ear. Seeing that others have similar struggles, and are surviving them, can make you feel less alone and less guilty.

As you accept the fact that you can't "do it all," it may become easier to build a support system to help you with day-to-day activities. Allow yourself to rely on family, friends, and neighbors who offer to help. If those in your immediate circle do not offer, then ask them for help. A relative who might be willing to babysit one evening a week can give you a much-needed respite. If you know other parents (single or not), offer to trade babysitting hours with them. Everyone needs breaks, not just single mothers.

If possible, involve the baby's father and paternal grandparents in child-care responsibilities. Even a newborn can have visitation with another parent, if that parent is responsible. If there are unresolved issues that would make this difficult, consider participating in some counseling with the baby's father. You will be parents together all of this child's life, even if you're never planning to live together. If you can communicate amicably, it can only be beneficial to the baby to be involved with both her parents.

It's important to involve your child with other men who are caring and responsive. Can your father, a brother, an uncle, cousin, or male friend step in on a regular basis? Having your child grow up with loving adults of both genders, regardless of the relationship, will foster his (or her) feelings of worth and self-esteem. And having other adults to share, even minimally, in the parenting burden will help you as well.

Grieving and anger.   Unless you carefully planned to become a single parent, you may have many unresolved feelings of loss or anger about your situation. You may need to spend some time working on those specific feelings about "what went wrong." Or you may feel disappointment about the elusiveness of the ideal Mama Bear, Papa Bear, and Baby Bear scenario. In either case, you need to allow yourself to pay attention to your feelings. It takes energy to push those feelings down inside you, and avoid feeling them; and you need to conserve all the energy you have right now. If you can let your feelings out and experience them, you can begin to accept your situation and move on to make the most of it. Single or married, you'll regret it later on if you don't have the most positive experience you can with your baby—because babyhood only lasts for an instant; then it's gone.

You may need to set aside time each day to cry, write out feelings, or rant and rave in front of the mirror. Talk into a tape recorder. Write letters and then tear them up. Give yourself permission to feel the way you do. You will likely find that you have more energy for other pursuits when you quit using so much energy to avoid your feelings. If you find that you just can't let go of the negative feelings about your situation, and they are coloring your relationship with your baby, it would be wise to talk to a professional therapist.

Make a structured plan.   Because the demands on your time are so great, getting everything down in a schedule is necessary. Map out all the things you need to do in a week. Pencil in work hours, child-care hours, and time for yourself. In the course of each day, you need some rest time, fun time, and contact with supportive adults. Single parents with outside jobs have reported that it works best to devote all their attention to the baby first thing after they work. Sit down and hold the baby, feed or rock the baby, play peek-a-boo. Spend at least 20 minutes focusing on the baby before you even change your clothes. You will feel less guilt if you know you've made an effort to build the parent-child relationship before you do anything else. Then you can move on to changing your clothes, fixing meals, and finishing the evening chores. Let the baby play in the crib or on the floor while you eat, take five minutes to shower, or refuel yourself in some other way. You not only gain some time for yourself, but your child will begin to develop some independence and the ability to calm or entertain himself. If your baby is fussy, rely on a front-pack or sling as you fix meals, pick up the house, or take your evening stroll.

The important thing is to make sure that you reserve, and *take*, some time for your own needs each day. If you can fit exercise, lunch with friends, and so on into your work schedule, this will be helpful. But, if not, reassure yourself about the need for you to make a schedule that includes time for your own recreation. Some single parents with calm babies find it helpful to use a kitchen timer, and to alternate the focus of their attention between the baby and other concerns. Set the timer for 20 minutes and play with the baby. At the end of that interval, set the timer for 20 minutes more and do something for yourself—after settling the baby in the swing, crib, or wherever she'll happily stay. Try alternating in this manner throughout the evening. Make sure you are not using all your 20-minute segments to wash dishes, vacuum, or fold laundry. The plan requires a healthy dose of fun and stress-relieving activities.

Important Note

If you find that putting the suggestions here (and in previous sections) into practice does not make you feel better, you may need to seek out a professional therapist. This is especially important if you fear that your resentment, anger, hopelessness, or other painful emotions may cause you to harm yourself or the baby. No matter how bad or hopeless your situation seems, you are not alone. Help is out there. Use the Resources Section at the back of this book for places to call if you need help right away.

6

Fathers And
Other Caregivers

The Short Version
(If You're Pressed for Time)

Chapter 6 is for dads. Now that your child is born, you may find
yourself in the midst of many significant changes, both in terms
of your emotions and your relationship with your wife. These
changes may come as a shock to you as the reality of fatherhood
sinks in. No matter how involved you were in your wife's pregnancy, you still may have felt like an "outsider looking in." You
may continue to have these feelings when everyone's attention
is focused first on the baby, then on your wife, and then maybe,
as an afterthought, on you.

   The goal of this chapter is to help you sort out whatever
feelings you have about all the changes in your life now. Take
our word for it—you are important, and your feelings have a major influence on your family's well-being.

Normal Changes of Fatherhood

   Just as new moms go through tremendous emotional and
relationship changes, so do new dads. You may find yourself ex-

periencing a wide range of emotions, from joy to uncertainty to anger. Even veteran fathers will go through these changes because of the physical and emotional demands that having a newborn presents. You may feel overwhelmed with providing for your enlarged family and assuming even more household responsibilities. You may feel left out and resentful of your wife's closeness with your child. At the same time, your life may seem richer now, and more fulfilled. All of these feelings are normal.

The Relationship Connection

It's crucial to keep in mind that changes in your partner's moods and behavior affect you, and vise versa. Remember those first few months of pregnancy when your partner's moods changed from one minute to the next? Déjà vu. Between sleep deprivation, your baby's feeding schedule, and all the physical and emotional demands of a newborn, you and your wife may feel exhausted and tense and, at times, dissatisfied with each other. Fortunately, infancy lasts a very short time. In the meantime, hold back and do not add any more responsibilities to those you already have outside your home. Help your partner with her postpartum physical and emotional recovery. Enlist all the assistance with child-care and household responsibilities you can find and afford.

If your partner is having physical or emotional problems that concern you, consult a health-care provider. Call your partner's obstetrician or the hospital where she delivered. Symptoms of postpartum depression and anxiety typically appear within the first two to three weeks following childbirth. Unlike the "baby blues," which are normal emotional changes accompanying childbirth, and which diminish as time passes, postpartum depression and anxiety get worse as the weeks go by. Postpartum thought disorders, which only affect 1 woman in 1,000, tend to occur within the first 24-72 hours after delivery. If your partner does not seem to be thinking clearly, or is hearing voices or having hallucinations, seek help immediately. Postpartum problems are very treatable if you get the right kind of help as soon as possible.

Getting Outside Help

As a man, you may have grown up believing that you should be able to fix all your problems on your own. It may make you feel incompetent or weak to think about asking for outside assistance. However, if your wife's difficulties are not improving

in spite of your efforts to make things better, you need to put your fears and reluctance aside. Your best way to help "fix" the situation is to help your wife locate competent and compassionate health-care professionals. Go with your wife if you can on her visits to her doctor or therapist. Learn everything you can about her difficulties, and how you can assist in her recovery. Support her doctor's or therapist's recommendations if they seem sensible to you, whether these involve medication for your wife or making sure that the two of you go out twice a month together.

Sometimes, it may take the outside perspective of a relative or friend to jog you into recognizing a postpartum adjustment problem. Be open-minded if your family or friends suggest that your wife needs help. Listen to what they have to say. Let them support you in considering what needs to be done. Be strong enough to admit that there may be a problem. Put your family's welfare before your pride.

Exercise
This One's for Dad

Imagine yourself walking down a long corridor with a suitcase. On the walls of the corridor are pictures of your family, friends, and others who have been important in your life.

As you walk along, reach deep inside your memory and recall the qualities of these individuals that most influenced you. Kindness. Compassion. Respect for your individuality. Persistence. A sense of humor. Toughness. Strength. Stop to look at each picture, and ask yourself, "What qualities did these people have that I want to have as a father? Which of their characteristics do I want to avoid?" Put only those pictures in your suitcase which you want to keep. Leave the others on the walls. If there are some people you want to remember but you don't want to imitate in your new life as a father, tear off just part of the picture—a twinkling eye or a strong, gnarled hand—to help you remember them.

If you did not have many positive influences from other people growing up, imagine how you would have liked your relationship with your own dad to have been. Create a scrapbook in your mind of the qualities you wish your dad had. Maybe being less strict. Or making time to play with you, instead of always working. Maybe just being a part of your life. Put this scrapbook in your suitcase, too. Use these pictures to guide you through your journey of becoming the father you want to be, and to assemble new snapshots of fatherhood for your children. Ones they will want to keep.

6

Fathers And
Other Caregivers

Like women, men go through enormous emotional and relationship changes following the birth of their child. If you're a new dad, you know this to be true. The problem is that little has been written about what dads go through, and few people talk about it. Who has asked you lately how you are? Chances are, most of the attention is focused on your wife and your baby. But that doesn't make the changes you're experiencing any less important or painful. After all, your world has been turned upside down, too.

In this chapter, you'll discover how normal it is to feel that your whole life has changed now that you have a baby. This may be especially true for first-time dads, but veteran fathers must also adjust to postpartum changes with each new child. We'll explore how your wife's postpartum adjustment may be affecting you, and we'll give you some guidelines about what to do if problems occur. Concerns and feelings that may interfere with either or both of you seeking help are reviewed; and we make suggestions about what you can do to overcome these obstacles. The chapter concludes with a discussion of how family and friends can approach you and your partner if they notice difficulties in your postpartum adjustment that you may have overlooked. Sometimes, an outside perspective may be what you need to get things back on track.

Your Baby Is Born

For months, you have stood by and watched while your wife's belly got bigger with the new life growing inside her. Although you probably felt the baby kick, or saw an ultrasound picture, the reality of having a child may have been difficult to grasp. For men, there is no tangible marker of fatherhood until the baby arrives. Then, in a split second, you go from cheering on the sidelines to receiving the quarterback snap. What a way to join the game! The team is charging ahead, and you aren't certain what play has been called. You may feel excited, confused, or scared. But one thing is certain—there's no turning back.

If you were present at your baby's birth, you probably experienced many different feelings. You may have been frightened by the pain your wife was in. You may have been amazed at all that went on. You may have gotten a little queasy. And yet, when your son or daughter popped out, you most likely felt a joy in your heart unlike any other you have known. You may have been so happy that you started to cry. Feelings of tenderness and caring may have welled up inside you.

All these feelings, whatever you experienced, are normal. So are the feelings of fear and uncertainty that may have set in later, as you wondered how you were going to care for this fragile new life. For both men and women, the responsibility of having a child, who depends solely on the two of you for his or her survival, can be intimidating, to say the least. Don't be alarmed. Over time, you will master this fatherhood game. But for now, take a deep breath and go slowly.

Just as women go through tremendous postpartum changes, so do men. Emotional ups and downs are part of normal postpartum adjustment. Remind yourself of this. Some men even experience physical changes along with their wife during pregnancy, putting on weight around the middle, or losing sleep at night while she tosses and turns and hoists herself out of bed every few hours to pee. One man we know pushed so hard during his wife's labor that he developed hemorrhoids!

You may not have given birth, but you are still faced with the daily demands and lifestyle changes that come with a new baby. You're woken up in the middle of the night, even though you have to go to work in the morning. If your wife is staying home to care for the baby, you may be doing double duty around the house when you come home from work, with cleaning, cooking, and laundry. You say you feel tired. Of course you do! Unfortunately, men are kept even more in the dark than women about what to expect when parenthood begins.

Most men have very little or no experience at all with newborn babies. It may come as a shock when you find that they don't even smile at you, and may not give even the slightest sign of recognition. And they look terrible! Who could ever imagine that such a tiny, limp-looking thing could make such a lot of noise? When you're tired and physically run down, it's easy to feel irritable, unhappy, and frustrated. This is a natural response to what may have been in many ways a nasty surprise. Remember the blissful parenthood you were led to believe awaited you? It's time to face reality.

Begin by cutting yourself some slack as you adjust to these changes. Time-outs are called in all major sports, so why not with fatherhood? Think about what absolutely needs to get done, and then leave the rest to take care of itself. Making certain that you and your wife rest as much as you can may be the major priority. Break household tasks down into smaller chunks. Pat yourself on the back for running one load of laundry or for unloading the dishwasher. Keep expectations about your work outside of the home reasonable. You may want to take some time off if you can. This is particularly helpful the first two to three weeks, during your wife's early recovery. Depending on the flexibility you have with your job, keep work-related demands to a minimum. Now is not the time to push for that promotion, or to reorganize your department. You will have time for these things later on. Follow the guidelines for making a survival plan outlined in Chapter 4 of this book.

If you're staying home to care for your baby, be certain to rest as you are able, and follow a healthy diet. Take regular breaks. Try to exercise. Find other dads and moms to talk to who are also staying at home. Parent support groups may be offered through your neighborhood elementary schools or local churches. Attend a child-care class. Get all the help you can from family and friends. Plan a night out for you and your wife once every two or three weeks. Although postpartum changes are unavoidable, there are many things you can do to make them less painful.

The "Odd-Man-Out" Syndrome

As a new dad, you may find yourself wondering, "Where do I fit in?" The old saying comes to mind, "Two is company, three's a crowd." With your wife's new relationship with your baby, you may feel like the odd man out. Because you haven't experienced the physical changes of pregnancy and childbirth, your wife has a head start on feeling involved. Socially and biologically, there's a stronger emphasis on the mother-child relationship than on the dad's role in a child's early life. Mother love is talked about more than father love. Family members and friends pay more attention to the new baby and new mother than to the new father. On television, in magazines, and in advertisements, pictures of moms and their babies appear much more often than pictures of fathers and their babies (although these are gaining a new popularity). So, what's a dad to do?

If you're feeling like an outsider looking in, there may be many reasons behind this. Ask yourself how much your feelings of uncertainty, or "not knowing what to do," may be getting in the way of feeling connected to your newborn. Are you at all afraid of intruding on your wife's relationship with your son or daughter? What is your wife communicating about how involved she wants you to be? Some women become very protective and territorial around a newborn, even excluding the baby's father to some extent. What did you learn from your dad about being a parent? What did you learn from society about father-child relationships? What kind of father do you want to be? Ultimately, this last question is the most important one. Despite what you've learned or thought about fatherhood in the past, right now is your opportunity to decide what you'll be like as a dad.

While you're struggling to figure out where you fit in your new family structure, you'll probably be expected to do more than usual to support your family's daily existence. In general, this may mean assuming or at least helping with some of the responsibilities at home that your wife used to manage. This can range from cleaning and doing the laundry to bathing the baby and fixing bottles to paying the bills. You'll feel like you're playing many different roles at once, some of which you may know next to nothing about. Although times are changing, not many men are known for their housekeeping talents. If you feel incompetent in any of these chores—and especially if your wife yells at you if you do them wrong—you're bound to feel a little confused and resentful. After all, you're trying, aren't you? You may not like what is happening, and may feel angry and frustrated. Things were so much simpler before. You knew who you were and what you had to do. Now you're not sure if you're catching or pitching or playing the outfield. It's no wonder if you feel a little insecure.

If you already shared household responsibilities with your partner before the baby was born, you'll probably adjust more easily to picking up the slack. This is not to say that it will be easy, even if you did *all* the housework and cooking before. There is much more work involved in caring for an infant than in any household without babies. But you'll be at an advantage if you're already an old hand at running the dishwasher and doing the laundry. You may even be the one staying home with your baby while your wife returns to work. Such arrangements are much more uncommon than the other way around, but they're not unheard of—and sometimes they work very well. But whether or not you're staying home, you're more likely now to see yourself and your wife as equal partners in parenting if you were equal partners in the household before you had a child. This will give you a head start on becoming an active and involved father, and promoting your family's well-being.

Many new fathers feel uncomfortable because their new family responsibilities do not fit with their ideas about being a man, and with their self-image in general. After all, "real men" don't wear aprons, and they certainly don't push vacuum cleaners with a baby on their hip. When you were growing up, you probably saw your mom doing most of the work at home, and your dad caring for other responsibilities. In fact, you may never have seen your dad do the dishes or make the bed or run a load of wash. Perhaps you didn't do too many of these things yourself before you and your wife had a child. What will your friends say if they find that you missed playing golf so that you could catch up on the laundry? How can you skip *Monday Night Football* to grocery shop? What will your boss do if you ask for time off to take your baby to the doctor? It makes sense that you may feel awkward and reluctant to challenge our society's traditional images of manhood. On the other hand, it's sort of exciting to be at the forefront of a revolution—and, as a modern dad in America in the '90s, that's exactly where you are.

Challenge yourself to create your own picture of fatherhood that includes everything you want to be as a dad, a partner, and a person. With each generation, men are becoming more and more involved in their children's lives, and the impact of this has been tremendous. Dads and children are happier and healthier as a result of becoming closer. Also, moms and dads seem to have a better relationship when dads take a more active role in parenting. Remind yourself that fatherhood, like motherhood, is a process. You don't bring your baby home from the hospital and automatically feel like a father. This takes time, and the feeling of "fatherliness" changes as your child grows. No parent is an expert from the start. So plan on making mistakes. Your partner will make mistakes, too. Part of your job as parents is to forgive yourselves and go on.

Just because you don't have breasts doesn't mean that you can't be just as nurturing a parent as your baby's mother. Babies need much more than milk to grow and thrive. They need love; they need patience. They need strength. If they have both a mother and a father with these qualities, they are very lucky indeed.

Be patient with yourself, and keep your expectations on a modest scale. Be mindful of even small successes. With experience, you will feel more competent and assured about your new role.

Three in the Bed

Nowhere may your baby's presence be felt more strongly than in the bedroom. If you find yourself "sitting on the bench" as you observe your partner and baby's relationship, in the bedroom you may feel as if you're sitting in the upper bleachers.

To begin with, you and your wife may not be sleeping together or going to bed at the same time these days. This may be due to nighttime feedings, the demands of breastfeeding, and scheduling differences, as each of you adjusts to your new responsibilities. If you're in bed together some of the time, chances are good that all you're doing is sleeping. And who wouldn't? Your wife may still be sore as all get-out from her stitches. And the fatigue people experience in caring for a newborn is enormous.

Just being able to get up in the morning and make it through another day is a mark of success.

It's especially important to understand fatigue as a crucial aspect of your partner's moods and behavior. You may have a long day at work; but if your wife is staying home initially to care for your child, her day is much longer and much more exhausting. Imagine spending your entire day feeding, burping, changing, holding, and comforting your newborn. Now imagine doing this for at least eight hours straight with no breaks. Even when the baby sleeps, you're still on duty—it's not as if you can take 15 minutes off to walk somewhere and have a cup of coffee. No one comes to relieve you, and you have no other adults to talk to. Plus, everywhere you look, there's work to be done: dishes unwashed, laundry to fold, nothing in the house for dinner—and look at that kitchen floor!

Whichever of you stays home, most everything you have to give will go to the baby. During the first few months postpartum, you may have little energy left for yourself or each other, and this can be very scary. Well—relax. This phase won't last forever. As time passes, you and your wife will spend less time meeting the baby's physical needs, and will have more energy for each other. Understanding and patience will go a long way toward keeping your marriage from wilting in the meantime.

Another factor that may be influencing your partner's relationship with you is her close physical contact with the baby. Especially with newborns, there is a great deal of physical care involved. Most new moms who stay at home spend their days feeding, holding, cuddling, rocking, and carrying their child. Such physical contact builds a sense of emotional closeness and affection. Having these needs partially satisfied in her relationship with the baby, your wife may seem more remote in her relationship with you. Even though this is part of the normal bonding process that occurs between moms and babies, it may aggravate your feeling of being the "odd man out." To make matters worse, your wife may not want as much touching or fondling, because she needs a break from physical contact after spending all day with the baby. At night, she's very likely to be much more interested in sleep than sex.

Put yourself in her shoes. Imagine you had spent the day with someone clinging to you. How physically affectionate would you feel after that clinging creature finally went to sleep? Think about it.

So, with these thoughts in mind, let's return to the bedroom to talk about sex—the act that brought your baby into the world. You say you don't remember what sex is, and when you do, you miss it terribly. Maybe you're ready to resume your physical relationship, and your partner isn't. Try to keep in mind how fatigued she is, or how desperately she may need a break from physical closeness. It isn't that she doesn't want you. Many women miss having an active sex life after childbirth as much as their partners do. But the constant demands of a new baby have to come first. At least, they do for a while. There is no way around this. If you have to wait a few more innings to get off the bench, sit tight. Before you know it, you'll be back in the game. It's even possible that renewed interest and a deeper feeling of commitment may enhance your sex life. It has been known to happen before.

Like your partner, you may experience some reluctance about renewing your sexual relationship. With the baby's arrival, you may feel as if there's a stranger in the house, and this can put a damper on lovemaking. You may not feel the same sense of privacy you did before. When you were a couple, you were free to spend your time as you pleased, lovemaking included. Now you practically have to make an appointment to spend time together. What a drag! No spontaneity. No sense of freedom. You are on your baby's schedule. How can you enjoy lovemaking when your child may wake up at any moment, demanding attention? Some couples swear that their child has a sixth sense about when the parents are about to make love!

Lack of opportunity isn't necessarily the only problem. Many men feel rather horrified at the changes in their wife's body postpartum. Maybe your wife is suddenly looking more like your (or her) mother than the woman you married. And what guy hasn't been taken aback by a completely unexpected spray of breastmilk in the throes of lovemaking? Jeez. You may feel as if your baby is "emotionally" in bed with you.

But hold on. Remind yourself that your life won't always be like this. When your baby is no longer a baby, your life may begin to seem almost normal again. Until that time it's important to discuss your feelings with your partner—although we'd strongly suggest that you refrain from making any negative comments whatsoever about her appearance. That's the last thing she needs now! If there are issues and challenges facing you that *aren't* appropriate to discuss with your partner, then find another new dad you can talk to, or spend some time talking to a counselor. It's just as important for you to deal with your feelings as it is for your wife to deal with hers.

Although you may think most often about changes in your sex life, what you may be missing more are the feelings of closeness and affection you and your partner shared. Because your baby consumes so much physical and emotional energy, you may have little left for each other. This can be very unsettling. In response to these changes, you may feel rejected, neglected, unloved, or all of the above. You may feel angry and resentful that your newborn has come between you and your wife. You may feel betrayed and sad over this unexpected loss, and may even question why you wanted to have a child—or why you agreed to have a child—in the first place. This can be true even if you feel great tenderness and affection as you watch your wife with your baby. Perhaps you feel frustrated over how your life is different now, and long for it to be the way it was. You may wonder when you will feel like a couple again. When will it be your turn? Be patient. That time will come.

In the meantime, make certain that you and your partner spend at least 10 to 15 minutes every day talking together. What you say is relatively unimportant. The idea is that you are letting each other know that your relationship still matters. Once you have the energy and the confidence, find a sitter so that you and your partner can go out together every two or three weeks. Don't wait until six months or a year has passed. Many couples start having problems after their first child's birth because they stop talking and spending time together. Yes, time and energy may be scarce; but your relationship is the foundation of your personal and shared emotional well-being. Don't forget this. Set time aside to listen to each other, to review the feelings you're having about your new life. Try to understand your partner's situation, and what it feels like, as often as possible, but especially at times when you're feeling frustrated, hurt, or angry. Try to express your feelings in words rather than "acting out" or sulking. When your partner criticizes you for your way of dealing with the baby, keep in mind that she's speaking out of a biologically programmed protectiveness for your child. Babies benefit from the difference in styles between their mother's and father's way of handling them—even though it can be painful for the parents as they work on accepting those differences and coming up with compromises.

The most practical and productive approach you can take is to arrange what time you and your partner can share alone together, but to also find ways to feel close together *with* your child. Go on walks together, take a dip in a pool together, play "This Little Piggy" with one of you on each foot. Become special to each other even though you have a baby, and work to keep it that way.

The Couple Connection

Remember those first few months of pregnancy, when your partner's mood changed from one minute to the next? You may have felt like a human tennis ball, slammed from one hard surface to another, being spun in all sorts of different directions. Well, now you're back on the court, being bounced around even harder and faster. This is partly because of the changes your wife is going through with her postpartum physical and emotional adjustment. But it's also because of the changes you're going through with *your* postpartum adjustment. Changes in your partner's moods and behavior affect you, and vice versa—which complicates the situation even more.

A lot of men claim that their partner's feelings and moods don't affect them—that they can shut them out, and go merrily along. But, in all honesty, is it really humanly possible to do this? No matter how hard you try *not* to be affected, you'll feel differently depending on whether you're greeted with a warm smile and a hug or a sour and angry stare.

Unfortunately, the enormous demands of having a newborn can make even the most naturally cheerful people act and sound like the Wicked Witch of the West. When you feel physically and emotionally drained, it's all too easy to become irritable, angry, and out of sorts. And since it doesn't make sense to get angry at the baby, it's all to easy for you and your partner to direct these feelings at each other.

One first-time dad commented, "Every evening when I came back from work, it was a war zone. My wife would assault me at the door with how rough her day had been and how miserable she felt. She would yell at me for being able to get away from all this by going to work. It didn't matter if I'd had a good or bad day. She wouldn't ask, and didn't seem to care. All I heard about was how bad her life had become. Sometimes she would break into uncontrollable sobs.

"Then, before I could say anything, she would shove the baby in my arms, and walk away. If I mentioned that I was tired and needed a break, she exploded about how selfish and thoughtless I was. She told me that I had no idea what it was like to stay home. She said that I didn't want the responsibility of having a baby, just the fun. After a while, I started staying later at work. I didn't want to come home to her fussing and putting me down. The more I stayed away, the more unhappy she became. But at least when I was gone, I didn't feel so bad."

Although this is an extreme example, some of it may sound familiar to you. The point is that your partner's feelings and actions affect you, and your feelings and actions affect her. Also, the increased pressures and demands of having a baby may naturally lead to greater conflict, because each of you feels more stressed and run down. As personal frustration and unhappiness build, you may feel more negative toward your partner. In turn, she may respond more negatively to you. Typically, this results in more fighting and disagreements, or more distancing and avoidance of each other. Sometimes, the way couples deal with conflict is to pull further away until there is little or no relationship left. Despite a lack of open fighting, this response can be equally damaging to a marriage or partnership.

On the other hand, having a child can deepen the positive feelings that couples share. To see your partner holding your newborn may stir strong feelings of love and tenderness in you. To watch her rocking or soothing your baby may intensify your feelings of caring and compassion. To see each other filled with pride and joy at the new life you've created may bring you closer together. While you watch each other struggle through the changes and trials of parenthood, you may develop a deeper understanding and commitment to each other. This can bring about a stronger realization of your ability to face life's challenges and grow from them, and a greater appreciation for what each of you has to offer personally, and what a strong team you can be.

Your Family's Well-Being

Although you can't totally eliminate postpartum stresses, there are some things you can do to improve your postpartum adjustment. The most important of these is to make yourself and your family your top priority for now. Initially, concentrate on the basics—sleeping enough, eating healthily, exercising, and spending time with your partner and child. This may mean temporarily suspending some of your other activities from the outside. Perhaps you'll bowl once a week instead of twice, or golf every other weekend instead of every Sunday. It may mean attending fewer professional association or club meetings. It may mean accepting fewer new responsibilities at work, if you can avoid them. In one way or another, taking care of yourself and your family will probably require staying home more and going out less. Your immediate family needs you right now more than outside friends, extended family, business associates, and acquaintances.

Infancy doesn't last long, but it's a critical time in your family's life. And because of the physical and emotional demands involved, neither you nor your partner can afford to get run down. So, put your energy into caring for yourselves and your baby. Do what you can to see that each of you sleeps and eats adequately. If one of you requires less sleep than the other, let that partner stay up later with the baby. Alternate nighttime feedings so that each of you gets one solid block of sleep. Sometimes breastfed babies can be supplemented with a bottle at night without disrupting their breastfeeding. If not, do what you can to relieve your partner of other physical responsibilities, like laundry or housework.

Always keep in mind that your partner's physical and emotional recovery will affect *your* postpartum recovery. The better she feels, the better you will feel. Working with your partner, prioritize what tasks at home are most important to complete. First make certain that your basic needs are met. Once this is done, choose one or two small goals for each week. These could be as basic as doing a few loads of laundry or cleaning the bathroom. Keep your expectations modest. Don't expect to spend a whole weekend working in the yard. Suspend any remodeling projects you may have. If you have some extra energy, maybe you and your partner can go out. If you can't go out, stay home and relax together. Talk frequently about how things are going, and what each of you can do to help the other.

Besides taking these steps, see that you and your partner get regular breaks from child-care responsibilities. Let family and friends do all they are willing to do. Having someone else fix a meal or hold the baby can provide much-needed relief. You might get half an hour to put your feet up, take a nap, or be with your partner. Don't worry that your helpful friends are doing too much. Right now, you and your partner are the ones who need a break. And if friends and family haven't volunteered their assistance, don't be shy about asking. They'll say no if they want to. In the meantime, speak up about what you need, even if this means letting your helpers know when you need a break from *them*. Be sure to limit the number of visitors you have over during the first few weeks your baby is home. This will aid your recuperation. If you feel awkward telling friends who drop by that this just isn't a good time to visit, keep a ratty T-shirt and pair of old slippers by the door. Slip these on before you answer the door to let your visitors know that they need to come another time, after you've had some sleep.

If you don't have family and friends to rely on, you and your partner need to make a schedule for giving each other "time-outs." See that each of you gets two to three hours a week to do whatever you want. This may not seem like much of a break, but it's still enough time to recharge. Although halftime passes quickly, the players still feel more energetic when they resume the field. Use your breaks wisely. Don't run around trying to get things done. You'll regret it when you're back on duty. Instead, put your feet up and read the paper. Watch something you enjoy on TV, or watch a funny video. Go out running or for a bicycle ride. Walk out in the garden and sniff the flowers. Let yourself unwind. Indulge yourself by just doing nothing. You've earned a rest.

Determining Whether Your Partner Needs Professional Help

Normal postpartum adjustment presents enough challenges. But between 10 and 20 percent of all women experience postpartum depression and anxiety. About 1 in 1,000 women will experience a postpartum thought disorder or psychosis. Postpartum problems can be very scary, frustrating, and unsettling, especially because they occur at a time in your life when you expect to feel so happy. After all, having a baby is supposed to be joyful, not troubling. If your partner has postpartum depression or anxiety, you may find yourself thinking over and over again, "It wasn't supposed to be like this."

Symptoms of postpartum depression and anxiety typically appear within the first two to three weeks following childbirth. Unlike the baby blues, which are time-limited changes in mood primarily due to the hormone changes of labor and delivery, postpartum depression and anxiety get worse as the weeks pass.

Postpartum thought disorders tend to occur within the first 24-72 hours following childbirth. If you have any suspicion that your partner has a thought disorder—if she's not thinking clearly at all, has lost touch with reality, or is very "speeded up" (in other words, has postpartum mania), seek help immediately. Don't put off phoning your wife's doctor, or taking her to the emergency room if need be (be sure to line up some-one to watch the baby while you're gone). Postpartum thought disorders can actually pose a threat to your partner's life, or that of your baby. Prompt medical assistance is absolutely necessary.

For an explanation of postpartum adjustment problems, from the baby blues to thought disorders, refer to Chapter 2. Your partner's symp-toms may not fit exactly into one diagnostic category. Anyway, unless you're a trained helping professional, you can't expect to come up with a diagnosis yourself. What you *can* do is to notice whether her symptoms are disrupting your daily lives, or keeping her from caring for herself or the baby. If that's the case, she should get professional care to keep her symptoms from getting worse.

Remember, your partner is not to blame for her difficulties, nor are you. Use the information in Chapter 2 to try to sort out what kind of help the two of you may need. This can be a frustrating, terribly painful time for you, and it's easy in this situation to lay the blame at each others' feet. But neither one of you is to blame. Blame it on hormones. Then get help if you need it, right away.

Being Able To Admit There's a Problem

Keith and Lisa had been married for two years when they decided to have a baby. Both high-powered career people, they never imagined that having a child could create any major problems for them. They were eager to start a family, and to master this new domain. But four weeks after their son's birth, Lisa went into a tailspin. She was so nervous, she couldn't sit still, and cried frequently. She began having panic attacks dur-ing which her heart raced and she felt light-headed. A few times, she actually passed out. She had no confidence about how to care for the baby. She became so afraid of being alone that she didn't want Keith to go to work. Every day, she would stand at the door and beg him not to leave. Then, she collapsed, sobbing as his car pulled away.

Keith couldn't believe this was happening to her. "Lisa was always such a strong person. I felt like I didn't know her anymore. I kept telling her to pull herself together, to work harder at feeling better. But she couldn't. She only got worse. Whenever she talked about getting outside help, I said we didn't need it—that, together, we could work things out. I wanted us to be self-reliant. I guess I felt like a failure not to be able to "fix it" ourselves. By the time Lisa saw a psychologist, she almost had to be hospitalized. And I still thought she could get over it without help. I couldn't admit how much trouble we were in."

Feelings like Keith's about his wife's postpartum difficulties are fairly common. If your partner is experiencing a postpartum reaction, you may be feeling frustrated that the two of you can't "fix it" on your own.

Growing up, you may have been taught that a "real man" can fix any problem if he tries hard enough. You may not want to face the reality of your partner's symptoms. You may want to pretend that things are "okay" or not "that bad." This is not because you don't care, but most likely a way of stopping yourself from feeling overwhelmed and frightened. It's very scary to see your wife acting so unlike herself. You may be worried about the added responsibilities this places on you. You may be angry over what is happening. You may feel that you ought to be able to make things right, that you're powerless to do so. You may wonder when your life will ever be normal again. Underneath everything, you may feel helpless and at a loss, wondering, "What do we do now?"

As a result of these feelings, you may pull away from your wife to lessen the pain. You are not being cowardly. Who wants to stand there and have salt poured into an open wound? As a way of coping, you may withdraw into your work or some leisure activity you enjoy. You may spend less time at home. Although withdrawing from your partner may help you feel better, the problem is that it may actually make her postpartum reaction worse. The less supported and cared for she feels, the more likely she is to continue to have problems. If a new mom feels that her partner is "hanging in there with her," she has a much better chance of a rapid postpartum recovery. Hanging in there may be more challenging than hiding, but in the long run it will make you a stronger team.

Your partner's postpartum difficulties may influence how you feel about your child. You may regret your decision to become a parent or have another child. You may have second thoughts about the timing of having this baby. You may resent your child, and blame him/her for your partner's problems. Of course, you know deep down that he/she isn't responsible, but it's hard to think clearly when your whole life seems to be going up in flames. You may avoid playing with your child, withdrawing as you have from your partner. Or you may become the primary caregiver, because your partner can't cope with child-care responsibilities now. This may strengthen your feelings of love and affection for your baby. However you respond, be patient with yourself. Your partner may be experiencing the symptoms, but you are going through a difficult time, too. No, it wasn't supposed to be like this. So, take a deep breath, acknowledge your feelings, and read on.

Getting Help

Before things get even more out of hand, it's time to take some action. Even though you may feel as if your partner's problems will never improve, this is not the case. Postpartum reactions are very treatable if you get the right kind of help. There is no reason for the two of you to keep on suffering. Something can be done, whether this means working together on different ways to manage postpartum changes, joining a support group for couples with postpartum problems, or consulting a professional health-care provider. In some situations, professional help is definitely needed. Don't criticize yourself because you can't "fix it" on your own. Admitting that you need help is a sign of strength, not weakness. It would be foolish to limp around on a broken leg, wouldn't it? Think of your postpartum problems as an injury that needs to be treated.

Jim had always prided himself on getting things done on his own. At 17, he left home and began supporting himself. He worked every summer, and half-time during the year, so that he could put himself through college. By 35, he had worked his way up to a partner in a prestigious engineering firm. With his future secured, he and Sandy, his wife of three years, decided it was time to start a family. Both of them were thrilled. Jim had worked so hard to get ahead. Now he could look forward to savoring his success with Sandy and his new family.

Within six months, Sandy was pregnant. Despite occasional bouts of nausea and insomnia, her pregnancy went smoothly. The nine months passed quickly, and Jim never felt happier than the day he drove his wife and their new son home.

For the first few weeks, things were fine. Then Sandy lost her appetite and couldn't fall asleep at night. Instead, she would lie in bed thinking about everything she had to do the next day. When she got up the next morning, she was nervous and depressed. Some days, she refused to get out of bed at all. Jim tried to reason with her, but it didn't work. He reminded her that both of them wanted this baby, and pleaded with her not to act this way. It seemed to Jim as if all his dreams were shattering and he didn't know where to turn or what to do.

Over the next few weeks, Sandy developed more symptoms. She became irritable, moody, and withdrawn from their son. This really upset Jim. "I couldn't understand her not wanting to hold our baby. We had both wanted this child more than anything. Feeling desperate, Jim phoned Sandy's obstetrician, who said that he thought she might have postpartum depression. The words "postpartum depression" frightened Jim, because he had never known anyone with a "mental illness." At the suggestion of Sandy's OB, he phoned a psychologist who specialized in postpartum reactions. "This was the hardest step to take—admitting to a total stranger that something was terribly wrong."

If you think that your partner's postpartum reaction is likely to require professional help, skip to Chapter 7 for guidelines on what to do. As a rule of thumb, the greater the number of symptoms, and the more they are interfering with your daily lives, the more important it is for you to seek professional help immediately. If your partner's symptoms have lasted longer than six weeks postpartum, and are not improving, consult a health-care professional who is knowledgeable about postpartum reactions. Don't wait because you hope things might get better on their own. The sooner the two of you get help, the quicker your situation will improve. Like an injury, postpartum episodes are easier to treat in the early phases than when secondary complications set in.

If your partner's symptoms aren't keeping her from caring for herself or the baby, and you are uncertain about the kind of help you need, there are some things you can do on your own to help. Read the symptom checklists in Chapter 2, and make a check mark by each symptom you've noticed in your partner. Then turn to Chapter 4, and read our suggestions about what the two of you can do for each symptom (there's a symptoms index at the beginning of that chapter). Follow these recommendations for a week or two. At the end of that time, look at whether her symptoms have changed. Are they better or worse? Have any gone away altogether? Have any new ones appeared? Overall, how does your partner say she feels? How do *you* think she is doing? If the two of you agree that things are improving, follow the suggestions in Chapter 4 to try to relieve her remaining symptoms for another week or two. Then reevaluate. If you think there has been no improvement, or if things are worse, read in Chapter 7 about getting professional help.

Problems with Getting Help

David's son was ten months old when he and his wife, Jane, decided to get help for her postpartum adjustment problems. Jane had done fine the first few months of Zach's life, but once she returned to work and stopped breastfeeding, she felt more and more depressed and anxious. Crying spells gave way to days of blue moods to weeks of feeling down. At about six months postpartum, she began having panic attacks, which made her afraid to drive most places on her own. David tried to be patient, but couldn't understand why going grocery shopping had suddenly become such an ordeal. He kept encouraging Jane to do more things on her own, despite her insistence that she couldn't.

By nine months postpartum, Jane was having trouble getting out of bed in the morning. She would complain of headaches, nausea, and dizziness. She often had David drive her to work, because she was afraid of her anxiety overcoming her on the way there. Jane's friends suggested she see a psychiatrist, but she and David were reluctant to go because "only crazy people do that." David recalls, "I never had anxiety or depression, so I didn't know how bad it could get. My father had a sister who cracked up after her last child was born, and spent the rest of her life in an institution. That scared me to death. I thought they might want to put Jane away or give her shock treatments. I couldn't let that happen."

Finally, a good friend of Jane's, who had experienced postpartum depression, persuaded them to go see her doctor. "I couldn't believe I was going to see a shrink," admitted David. "I didn't know how he could help us. I was so frustrated and down on myself, I didn't think anything could help."

The doctor explained that postpartum depression affects 10 to 20 percent of all women. Jane and David weren't alone—many couples have to face this nightmare that no one talks about. Part of Jane's problems had to do with physical changes she experienced after Zach's birth. To correct this, the doctor put her on some medicine. "That shook me up all over again. How bad could this be? Still, we listened and followed his instructions. We also saw a counselor who helped us make other changes, and discuss what we were going through. I never expected any of it to work, but six months later, our life was much better. Twelve months later Jane was off all her medicine and things seemed pretty normal. I feel that getting professional help saved our family. I will always be grateful for this."

If your partner is having a postpartum reaction, you may be hesitant to see a psychiatrist or psychologist because of the stigma. Although times have changed, the attitude persists that you have to be "nuts" to talk to a mental health provider. As mentioned earlier, admitting that you need outside help may be another obstacle for you. After all, weren't you always taught to keep going, even if you were in terrible pain—to tough it out, never let them see you sweat; never let them see you cry? It may go against everything you've ever been taught about being a man to ask for help now.

The problem is that almost every man needs help at some time in his life. Considering what you and your partner have been going through, getting the help you need is a perfectly logical and reasonable thing to do. A competent mental health provider can evaluate your situation, and make suggestions about different measures you can take to help your partner feel better and get your situation back to normal.

Of course, no one ever expects to need help from a psychologist or psychiatrist. But being wise enough to admit your need is a sign of strength, not weakness. It would be foolish for a diabetic not to take insulin because she was determined to defeat her diabetes on her own. And how useful or kind would her partner be acting if he supported her in going without the medication? Try to think of postpartum reactions in the same way. If you broke your arm, you would go to a doctor to have it set. With problems involving your family's emotional health, a psychologist or psychiatrist is the right kind of doctor to see.

Another difficulty with seeking help may be that it makes the uncomfortable feelings you are experiencing even more real. It's one thing to admit to yourself that you're feeling fearful, powerless, or inadequate to make things better—this may be troublesome enough. But to think about sharing these feelings out loud with a mental health provider, or anyone else—forget it! You already know that your life is falling apart, so what can you possibly gain from talking about it?

What you may not realize is that mental health providers, because of their expertise, may offer other solutions than what you have considered on your own. As an outsider looking in, they will have a different perspective than you or your wife, and this can be immensely helpful. While you are quarterbacking the game, they are standing on the side-lines, where they can view the playing field as the action unfolds. Like a skilled coach, they can help guide you to the goal line; but this will require your best effort and willingness to work together.

Asking for help may challenge your belief that talking about painful things will make a bad situation worse. Many men are still puzzled over why their partners feel better just talking about their problems rather than taking action to fix what is wrong. Be patient. Usually, some combination of talking and action is required. Experiment with discussing your thoughts and feelings. See what happens. Cooperate with new sugges-tions. Trust your health-care provider to call the plays, and if his or her coaching isn't working out, then speak up. Your input is important. It's your family's emotional well-being at stake. Remember that progress in-volves two steps forward, and one step back. Give yourself and your partner time to heal. Make your family's recovery your top priority, and stick to it.

A third obstacle in getting help may be that you don't know where to find it. If your partner is experiencing a postpartum reaction, you may feel frustrated over not knowing a health-care provider who specializes in these problems. In many smaller communities, there may be a lack of qualified professionals. But don't be discouraged—help is out there, al-though it may take a little work to find the right provider.

To begin with, contact your partner's obstetrician, and ask for a reference to a psychologist or psychiatrist who is knowledgeable about postpartum adjustment problems. If the OB doesn't know someone ap-propriate, phone the hospital where you delivered, and speak to someone in the childbirth education department about a referral. You can also con-tact your local mental health association or clinic, and inquire about some-one with expertise in this area. If you or your partner know someone—or know *of* someone—who had a postpartum reaction, make contact and ask about her experience with local providers.

Another way to find a professional helper is to call Depression After Delivery (DAD) at 1-215-295-3994 or 1-800-944-4PPD. DAD is a national organization founded to assist families with postpartum problems. They publish a national directory of postpartum health-care specialists, as well as a listing of postpartum support groups in the United States. If you learn of a support group in your community, you can phone the contact person there and request a referral to a qualified specialist. Women who have been successfully treated for a postpartum reaction may be the best equipped to offer a recommendation. If none of the previous suggestions yields a referral, find the agencies in your community that work with moms and families, and continue your search. If you live in a *very* remote community, you may have to "commute" to therapy; or you might even choose to stay with friends or family—or in a motel—in another town where qualified help is available. In cases of a severe postpartum reaction, you and your partner may choose an inpatient facility as the most practical place for her recovery.

Do not give up the search. Help *is* available. Keep looking until you find someone who is experienced and competent. And if you aren't satisfied with the first person you find, look further. For additional information about seeking help from a mental health professional, turn to Chapter 7.

No, Not Medicine

If your caregiver recommends putting your partner on medication, the idea may be as disturbing to you as was seeking help in the first place. You may see taking medicine as a sign of weakness, or a failure on your part, to beat this problem on your own. Many men and women will endure high levels of physical pain before taking a single aspirin. The idea of having to be on psychiatric medicine to cope with anxiety and depression is particularly unappealing. Chances are, your partner has her own reservations. When you add your concerns to hers, problems can quickly develop.

Janet sought professional help six weeks postpartum because of uncontrollable anxiety. She couldn't sit still for longer than five minutes at a time. She had hot flashes, a racing heart, and felt totally unable to care for her infant son. She thought she was losing her mind. Against her husband's wishes, she consulted a psychologist who specialized in postpartum reactions. The psychologist referred her to a psychiatrist, who put her on anti-anxiety medication, and instructed her to take it daily. Janet didn't want to take the medicine, because she was afraid of becoming dependent on it, and saw needing medicine as a failure. But she reluctantly agreed to follow her doctor's advice.

At first, she hid the medicine from her husband, Bob. She knew he wouldn't understand and would give her a hard time about it. She could barely deal with her own feelings of inadequacy and self-contempt. Then, one day, Bob discovered the medicine in Janet's purse when he was looking for her car keys. "I was really disgusted," he recalled. "I thought it was bad enough that she had gone to see a psychiatrist. I told Janet she didn't need to be on medication, and that we could work this out together. I know she felt ashamed because of what I said, but I couldn't stop myself. I felt so lousy about her taking medicine and having problems. I just kept thinking, we can do this on our own. We don't need any crutches—any doctor or medicine. We can do it alone."

After Bob's discovery, Janet stopped taking her medication. During the next few days, her anxiety became almost unbearable. She kept pacing the floor while the baby lay in the crib nearby, crying to be fed. She could not stop wringing her hands, and seemed to be losing touch with reality. Bob felt bad, and called her doctor to report what had happened. The doctor discussed Bob's reluctance to see Janet on medication. Bob wasn't alone, the doctor explained; many men react negatively to the idea of psychiatric medications. But, in Janet's case, she needed medicine to get better. The doctor reviewed the physical aspects of having a postpartum anxiety reaction, and how the medicine would relieve Janet's symptoms. Once Janet's anxiety level was lowered, she'd be better able to care for the baby. The doctor emphasized the importance of her staying on the medication as long as necessary, and continuing in counseling to aid her emotional recovery.

While Bob still didn't like the fact that Janet needed medicine, he was convinced by the doctor of the importance of her taking it, and was able to support Janet in following the doctor's advice. Within 24 hours of resuming her medicine, Janet felt better. Nine months later, she experienced full recovery, and was able to get off of the medicine without a relapse.

If you're feeling worried or concerned about your partner being on medicine, speak with her doctor. Don't advise her on your own to stop taking it. Some medicines are dangerous to quit cold turkey, and may cause withdrawal symptoms. Find out why the doctor feels that it's necessary for her to be on medication. Ask what kind of symptom relief is expected, and how soon. Watch for signs of improvement. If you don't notice any change for the better, consult the doctor again. Some medicines take longer to work than others. The doctor may need to try a few different medicines before finding the right one. Take an active role in your partner's recovery by going to the doctor with her and reporting your observations. Inform yourself about the known side-effects of her medication, and watch for these.

Above all, keep an open mind. Remember—right now, your partner may need psychiatric medication to be well in just the same way in which a diabetic needs insulin. Don't judge her or yourself harshly for being unable to "fix" her postpartum problems on your own. For more information on psychiatric medicine, see Chapter 7.

Surviving Postpartum Changes

Whether problems develop or not, having a child results in enormous emotional and relationship changes. Keep this in mind as you encounter the ups and downs of fatherhood. Refer back to this chapter and read Chapter 4, for ideas about what to do to improve your postpartum adjustment. Remember to make your family's physical and emotional well-being your top priority. Take care of yourself by resting, eating a balanced diet, taking breaks from child-care responsibilities, and keeping your expectations and goals small. Let family and friends help as much as they're willing, and let them know how you want things done.

If problems occur, follow the suggestions in this chapter to determine what kind of help is needed. Don't hesitate to seek outside help if it is required. The sooner you receive help, the quicker your situation will improve. Don't let any concerns you may have about consulting a health-care provider get in the way. Remind yourself that if you had a broken leg it would be foolish to limp around on it without having the bone set, and risk crippling yourself for life. The same wisdom holds true when it comes to dealing with postpartum reactions. To admit when you can't fix something on your own is a sign of wisdom, not weakness. Be open-minded if family and friends suggest that there may be problems that neither you nor your partner have recognized. Listen to what they have to say. See if it fits your perceptions. If it does, think about what needs to be done.

Don't expect yourself to have all the answers—no one does. But by setting aside your fears, you may stop your partner's postpartum difficulties from getting worse, and put your family back on the road to recovery.

From the Sidelines:
Some Gentle Advice for Family and Friends

Because of all the changes you and your partner are experiencing, the two of you may not be in the best position to notice problems if they occur. This is another area in which family and friends can be especially helpful, just as it's easier to see the whole playing field from the sidelines than as a significant player in the game. Although other family members and close friends may be involved with helping you as you adjust to your life with a new baby, they are still likely to have a different perspective than you and your partner.

If you're a relative or friend who has noticed problems developing, consider taking the following steps. First, approach the new parents in a direct but noncritical way. Let them know that you understand they are doing their best in meeting the many challenges of caring for a newborn. If you are a parent yourself, relate some of the difficulties you experienced. Let them know that they aren't alone. Help them not to feel like failures. Be specific about the changes or problems you've observed that are concerning you. It may be easier for them to relate to concrete examples of what you see as problematic. Just saying, "You seem unhappy," or "You seem upset," may not be enough. Ask them what they think about your observations. Try to get both partners to share their reactions, and discuss what you've said.

Next, assist the couple in thinking about what may need to change for their situation to improve. Offer to contribute your time and energy as part of the solution, if you can realistically do this. Discuss other resources they might use. For example, if the new mom is getting distressed because she has no relief from child care, explore which family members and/or friends could come over during the week to lend a hand. Find out the days or hours when a babysitter would be most welcome and offer to contact friends and set up a schedule for the next few weeks. You might be able to arrange for these same well-wishers to deliver a hot meal a few times a week, or even every night for a week or so. Or if the new parents have the money, you might suggest that they hire people to help out with housework, shopping, cooking, and child care. If money isn't that abundant, there may be a teenager in the neighborhood who would work after school for a modest wage and help with some of the chores or just watch the baby. Even an hour of help a day can be of tremendous value to a new mother. Be creative in reviewing all the possibilities. Encourage the couple to start with what they think will work best for them. Applaud them for being willing to look for solutions.

If you think the new parents need professional help, let them know this. Use tact in the way you present them with this idea, but be direct and be honest. Explain your reasoning, noting the problems you've observed.

Be prepared for them to react with some discomfort, even to get angry with you. This is a difficult suggestion for almost anyone to hear, probably because "requiring professional help" continues to be associated with "being weak" or "being crazy." Take their response in stride. Don't take it personally or strike back with anger. Remind yourself that you have their best interest at heart, whatever their reaction. Remember that sometimes the truth is a hard pill to swallow, especially when it means admitting that all is not well. Realize that it may take time for them to accept what you've said.

If they do decide to seek professional care, help them find someone who is experienced and competent. Ask other people whom they would recommend. Look for someone who has a proven track record of successfully treating postpartum adjustment reactions. If a person with postpartum expertise is not available in your community, choose the individual who is regarded as the most skilled local provider of general mental health services.

Eileen was a 32-year-old attorney who was thrilled to be having her first baby. It had taken her three years to get pregnant, with the aid of infertility drugs. Carlo, her husband, vividly recalled how excited they were when her home pregnancy test came out positive. "I couldn't believe, after everything we'd been through, we were going to have a child. I felt so blessed. We spent months buying baby furniture, and arranging the nursery. Eileen would sit in the rocking chair and sing to her belly. I kept imagining how it would be to hold my son or daughter in my arms. What a great feeling."

After a prolonged labor and delivery, Eileen came home from the hospital with their baby daughter. Already feeling fatigued and run down, only the excitement of having a new baby seemed to sustain her. Usually upbeat and optimistic, she suddenly felt unhappy and discouraged much of the time. A good friend, Sandy, noticed these changes, and decided to speak to her. "I didn't know how she'd take it, but Eileen seemed to be less and less herself. She was withdrawing from her family and friends, and that wasn't at all like her. She sounded down a lot. That shocked me, because I was used to her pulling me out of a funk. I didn't want to see her get any worse. I felt I had to say something."

At first, Eileen was startled. She said that she was tired from taking care of her daughter, and that was what Sandy was picking up on. A month later, when nothing had improved, Eileen thought some more about Sandy's remarks. "I knew there was some truth to what she'd said. I knew I was having problems. That was such a change for me—it was scary. I could handle everything that came my way before. Why not now? I knew other women who'd recently had babies and they were doing okay." Finally, with Carlo and Sandy's support, Eileen went to see a psychologist. She almost cancelled her first appointment. "I felt so ashamed—but I learned it was all right to not be Superwoman, and to make the changes that helped me recover. I know Sandy took a big risk in talking to me. I owe her a lot for that."

Be certain immediately to address situations that may become life-threatening. If the new mom tells you that she's having thoughts about harming herself or her baby, insist that she seek professional help. Be willing to accompany her to the health-care provider's office, or set up the appointment—or both. Make sure her partner knows about these thoughts. Encourage her to speak with her partner if she hasn't already. If she's fearful of her partner's response, ask whether she'd like you or another third party to speak with him. As horrible as these thoughts may sound, keep in mind that sweeping them under the rug is much riskier than dealing with them openly.

If the new mom is acting psychotic—if she reports hearing voices, seeing things that aren't there, or seems out of touch with reality in other ways, notify her partner first; then, see that the couple obtains immediate medical attention. The new mom also needs professional help if her main symptoms are rapid speech, extreme restlessness and irritability, lack of appetite and/or insomnia, and what seems like boundless energy—in other words, manic symptoms. Because either of these conditions may rapidly worsen, persist in pushing the couple toward getting professional help. Both the baby's and the mom's life may be at stake.

With both postpartum psychosis and mania, medication and, sometimes, hospitalization are routinely required. If necessary, get other friends and family members to help get the couple into treatment. Remind yourself that the consequences of their not receiving medical attention may be fatal. So do whatever it takes. They will thank you later.

7

Beyond Self-Help: Consulting a Professional

The Short Version
(If You're Pressed for Time)

Although you can accomplish a lot by changing how you take care of yourself in the postpartum period, there are limits to what you may be able to do on your own. At some point, you may feel as if you've exhausted your own resources for helping yourself: you really want someone else to guide you through this rough time. Or perhaps someone important to you, such as your partner or a family member, feels that you need to get professional help. If you reach that point, take heart: *you are not a failure.* The stresses in your life right now have simply become unmanageable. It can take real courage to admit that you need some outside help, guidance, or support. Be proud of yourself if you have that courage. You are taking the first step.

You need to remember several important points when you embark on your search for a professional helper. First of all, *you are the consumer.* You need to trust your ideas about what you need now. If you do not feel comfortable either with a therapist or the therapist's recommendations for your recovery, trust your instincts. You may need to "shop around" before you find someone who fits your personality and needs. You *can* find someone you can trust, if you hang in there. Look for a therapist who will be a guide and a partner in your effort to feel better—not an authority figure or someone who in any way will treat you with scorn. You know yourself best, and you're the only person on earth who knows whether a particular suggestion or course of treatment feels right to you. Convey this knowledge to any therapist you're considering.

There are three main criteria to look for in selecting a therapist. The first, is that any helper you select should be both caring and understanding. Second, the therapist should have some knowledge and expertise about postpartum adjustment as a life transition. He or she should readily acknowledge that this is a tough time in your life primarily because you have a new baby. The therapist's plan for you should be to work through the symptoms of your postpartum adjustment before you tackle any problems from the past. Take this book with you, and share the ideas here with your therapist. Let him or her know if you've found the approach here to be helpful; and be explicit that you would like help in putting your self-care plan into action. Finally, the therapist you ultimately choose should have some standard credentials, such as licensure or registration as a psychologist, social worker, or professional counselor. There are detailed guidelines for judging these criteria in the full-length version of this chapter.

You need to know that therapy is not a cure-all and no therapist is a miracle worker. Therapists cannot wave magic wands and suddenly make you feel better. Recovery is hard work, and will likely include lots of talking about your feelings, experimenting with trying to do things differently at home, and maybe even feeling worse before you feel better. You will still need to take care of yourself in the ways we've outlined in earlier chapters. Therapy may take only several sessions, or it may take several months or longer. Ask the therapist for a treatment plan that will detail the course of action he or she envisions for your recovery. You should not be at all in the dark about this. And you have the right and responsibility to communicate your own ideas about what will and won't work for you. Every treatment plan is subject to modification.

Sometimes psychoactive medication can be an important part of a postpartum treatment plan. Needing medication does not mean that you are weak or crazy or a failure. Rather, medication of this kind is used to correct some chemical imbalance in your body which is probably responsible for your postpartum reaction. This is a temporary measure—it does not mean that you'll be on medication forever. There are antidepressant medications, anti-anxiety medications, antipsychotic medications, sleep medications, hormone treatments, and antimania medications. Many postpartum women who are having severe problems are treated with one of these drugs or a combination of several. Some medications work quickly, some take longer. Some may have troublesome side effects, while others do not. Only licensed physicians, such as obstetricians, psychiatrists, and family practitioners, can prescribe medications. If the therapist you choose cannot prescribe medicine, but feels that medication would help you, he or she will have to work in consultation with a medical doctor.

Medication is not always the answer or the appropriate treatment; but in some life-threatening situations, it is the only choice. You need to know that many medications are not compatible with breastfeeding, although there may be some that you can take safely while continuing to breastfeed. If you do not want to wean your baby so that you can take medications, or you do not feel for any other reason that medication is the right choice for you, you can tell your therapist that you want to try other interventions first. *You are the consumer.* There are only a couple of situations (i.e., mania and psychosis) in which medication is absolutely essential for your health and the health of the baby.

Exercise
Two Minutes for Yourself

Close your eyes. Imagine a TV screen in your head. There's one channel that gives you a blank screen. If the channel drifts, showing you negative thoughts and worries, grab that remote control; switch back to the blank screen.

When you can hold the blank screen in your head, try switching to a channel that shows you a positive image of yourself in your role as a new mom. See yourself on the screen, coping with your situation, feeling relaxed and calm; looking in control. Hold that picture in your head. Focus on it. Study it in more detail. This is a videotape you're watching now. Rewind it, look at it again. Put the controller on "pause." How do you feel about that person on the screen? Do you admire her? Is she doing a great job? That's you you're looking at—give yourself a pat on the back. Then take a few slow, deep breaths and return to your day.

7

Beyond Self-Help:
Consulting a Professional

Julia had a seven-week-old baby. For the past four weeks, she had been feeling extremely tired, tearful, and tense. On the advice of her physician, she'd been napping twice a day. Her doctor had also recommended an antidepressant, but Julia was breastfeeding. She didn't want to give up the nursing, and she was uncertain about taking medication. She really wanted to figure out how to feel better on her own. She had a good group of friends in the neighborhood, mothers with infants and older children, who were taking turns bringing the family meals and providing a shoulder to cry on. Julia's husband was still taking a night feeding every other night to give her a break. And for two weeks, she had been taking a brisk walk every afternoon around the nearby park, hoping that exercise would lift her spirits. She had even talked to three different phone volunteers from Depression After Delivery. But as Julia worked to put everyone's suggestions into practice, she found that she felt only minimally better. What more could she do? Where could she turn?

The Limits of Self-Care

Many women and their families find that taking care of themselves physically and emotionally can turn their symptoms around. But just as many find that, no matter how well they pamper themselves, they continue to feel worse. With each passing day and week, the anxiety, fatigue, tearfulness, and other symptoms lift briefly, only to settle in again like a fog blocking out all the sunlight. Some of this may be part of the usual "two steps forward, one step back" process of recovery; and postpartum emotions tend in general to fluctuate wildly. But there are limits to what self-care can accomplish in many situations.

A new mother may be feeling so badly that she cannot get organized enough to do what she knows would help her feel better. Or, as in Julia's case, she may work very hard at doing all the "right things," and still feel overwhelmed by her symptoms. These limits are simply a reality.

It's important to listen to those who know you well when you're trying to decide whether to seek outside help. It's equally important to trust your own judgment. You know yourself best. When weighing input from your family, friends, and partner, it's best to err on the side of getting help rather than persevering unsteadily on your own. In other words, if you feel you want to seek professional help, you should do so. By the same token, if someone close to you is greatly concerned, and is urging you to consult with a professional even though you feel you should keep plugging away on your own, it's probably a good idea to take their advice and seek help.

Certain aspects of your behavior may be clearer to your loved ones than they are to you. At times—and postpartum recovery is one of those times—you may not be able to see yourself as objectively as those around you can. If you go to a psychologist or psychiatrist at someone else's urging, you can take that person with you. Having them involved as much as possible can greatly reduce his or her anxiety about your state of mind. The helping professional may even be able to give reassurance that you're doing well tackling things on your own. The peace of mind that can come with such reassurances will be well worth the cost of an initial consultation. If it seems that a course of therapy, medication—or both—is indicated, then you've wisely put yourself in a position where you can get help without delay.

Here are some general guidelines about when professional help is probably your best alternative:

1. You've worked on your own as long as you feel you can on this issue. You simply feel that you need a different perspective to turn things around.

2. You fear that you may harm yourself, the baby, or any other person.

3. You're unable to sleep for more than three to four hours for several nights in a row, or have other significant sleep problems.

4. You have no interest in eating, or eating makes you feel sick to your stomach. As a result, you have eaten little in the past few days.

5. You are unable to take care of the baby or your own needs (dressing, grooming, eating) because of your symptoms.

6. You are experiencing manic or psychotic symptoms (you've "speeded up" or are out of touch with reality—hearing voices or having hallucinations).

7. You've worked hard on a self-care plan for at least ten days, and still feel overwhelmed by your symptoms.

8. A significant person in your life believes that it's essential for you to get help.

9. You are having panic attacks or anxiety symptoms which interfere with your daily activities.

10. You are having postpartum adjustment symptoms (crying, anger, fatigue, or hopelessness, for example) which are preventing you from running your life as you would like to.

11. You are at least six weeks postpartum and your symptoms are not lifting, but are staying the same or getting worse.

Elizabeth was a 42-year-old anesthesiologist. After 12 years of marriage, she and her husband made the decision to have a baby. It took 16 months of trying and aggressive treatment for infertility, before Elizabeth finally conceived. She was sure she'd be coasting downhill from that point on. In her third trimester, she interviewed nannies in anticipation of returning to her position at the hospital after her three-month leave.

Elizabeth had a relatively easy birth, and felt well afterwards. Her baby boy slept well, nursed well, and left Elizabeth wondering why the new mothers she'd known had done so much complaining. Sure, she was tired; but this was nothing compared to the many nights during her residency when she worked 18-hour shifts. Feeling a little bored at home, and with the nanny ready to start, Elizabeth returned to her busy schedule when the baby was only five weeks old. That was when everything began to change for the worse.

Elizabeth still nursed the baby at night, and expressed her milk at work in her office three times a day. She often felt tired, and her breasts leaked between pumpings. She was so exhausted when she came home from the hospital that she had little energy left for the baby. But when she was at work, she missed him terribly; she could think of nothing else. Elizabeth began to feel tortured by guilt. She was acquainted with only one other new mother at the hospital, a technician who was 15 years her junior. She had little in common with this woman, and didn't feel drawn to confide in her. Larry offered reassurance, and made arrangements so that Elizabeth could take several hours each Saturday to spend as she wished. But Elizabeth was at a loss; she didn't know what to do with the time. She ended up spending most Saturdays and half of Sunday sleeping. She felt ill, but wasn't able to identify any symptoms apart from fatigue.

After three weeks of this, Larry and Elizabeth had a serious discussion about her condition. They decided she should return to the exercise class she'd abandoned during her pregnancy out of fear of miscarrying. She got in touch with a local "working mothers" group, and made a commitment to attend their meetings.

During their meetings the next week, Elizabeth made an effort to get to the exercise class; but something always popped up that made it impossible to go. She woke up with a stiff neck one morning. Then there was an emergency at work she had to attend to. She wrote the date of the mother's group meeting on the wrong night in her calendar. Accustomed to thinking of herself as organized and competent, Elizabeth wondered what was happening to her.

Finally, after three more disorganized weeks, she broke into tears just before a routine procedure, and was so upset that someone else had to be called in to replace her. She sobbed for two hours in her office, and wouldn't let anyone in the door. Finally, the head nurse on the ward called Larry who came to take Elizabeth home. Before they left, one of Elizabeth's colleagues from labor and delivery sat down with her and expressed her concern. When she said that Elizabeth looked overwhelmed, Larry chimed in with his own concern. Elizabeth wasn't functioning well either at home or at work. Larry mentioned that she didn't seem to be getting much pleasure at all from the baby after striving all that time to conceive. Elizabeth, normally calm and articulate, could only respond by breaking into tears again. As Larry and the OB continued to talk, and Elizabeth continued to cry, it became clear that she needed more than exercise classes or mommies' groups to lift her out of her depression.

If you decide that seeking outside help is your best option, try not to question your choice. You've shown a great deal of strength in being able to say, "I need someone else's help now." It takes considerable courage to admit this. There's still an outdated notion in our society that attaches a stigma to mental health problems. Some people who don't know any better may consider it a sign of weakness to seek the help of a psychologist or psychiatrist. You may find yourself, or those around you, buying into this view. And yet it's simply a false view; scientists are making discoveries every day that confirm the connection between our body and mind. A biochemical imbalance that triggers depression or mania is no more something to be ashamed of then a biochemical imbalance that triggers diabetes. It's simply foolish not to get treatment—whether medication, talking therapy, or both—when you need it. If you've done what you can by yourself and still don't feel good, outside input is necessary. You are not a failure—you're simply human.

It can help to think about a psychologist or psychiatrist as a health partner, as Ellen McGrath suggests in *When Feeling Bad Is Good*. The person you consult will help you see what's missing, and give you tools to fill the holes. You need someone to point you in the right direction now, and give you a boost. But even a helping professional can't simply "fix" you. You'll need to contribute your own hard effort and perseverance— your willingness to feel better. Deciding to find someone to help you is your first move. Now you can look forward to having a skilled partner in your struggle, rather than facing the challenge of feeling better on your own.

The Search for a Professional Helper

Finding a person whom you can trust to help you through this delicate life transition may seem daunting at first. Where do you go? Who can you ask?

There are many qualified professionals out there. You need to think of yourself as a consumer, entitled to be treated with respect. As Dr. McGrath states, you are doing some of the most important shopping in your life. You want to find a person who is not only competent, but caring as well.

The first criteria you want to use when shopping for a therapist are competence, compassion, and specific experience dealing with postpartum transitions. It's important for the therapist to have an understanding of the postpartum period as a major life transition that's unique among other times in your life. Miriam Greenspan, author of *A New Approach to Women and Therapy*, stresses that a helping professional should connect with you out of compassion and respect. The therapist needs to have knowledge about the sources of your suffering. Without specific experience and/or training in postpartum issues, this caring connection is more difficult for the therapist to achieve.

For help in finding a therapist who is knowledgeable about postpartum issues, you may want to contact Depression After Delivery (DAD) or Postpartum Support International (PSI). The numbers for these organizations are listed in the Resources Section. Both organizations can give you names and numbers of therapists, but don't screen them either for ability or credentials. That job will still be up to you.

If you can't find a therapist in your area by contacting PSI or DAD, go to other sources for referrals. You may want to begin by asking other professionals you know if they can make a recommendation. Your OB, internist, clergyperson, or childbirth educator is often familiar with mental health professionals, and can give you referrals or ideas about where else to look. Local hospitals, mental health associations, or professional psychological organizations may have referral networks which you can use. Other new mothers or mothers of young children may know of professionals in your community who work with postpartum issues. Many health insurance plans can identify or recommend professionals who participate in their organization. Once you have several names, you can begin to contact these professionals by telephone for further evaluation.

Professional standards are the second group of criteria to consider when looking for a therapist to help you through this difficult time. There are national and state organizations that license or register therapists. Professionals who belong to these organizations must meet certain minimum standards of training and experience. This is still no guarantee of competence. But it's important to evaluate any potential therapist in terms of qualifications, and licensure or registration with a governmental body is one place to start. There's a list of these organizations at the back of this book, in the Resources Section, along with an explanation of the different types of helping professional you can choose from.

Your first talk with the therapist will probably be by telephone. If you only reach an answering service when you call, you can specify that you'd like to talk to the therapist first by phone before making an appointment.

It's quite natural to feel awkward when you first talk with a helping professional, whether by phone or in person. First of all, you're calling because you're in pain, and it may go against everything you've been taught to be vulnerable in front of a stranger. This may be a new experience for you, and you may feel self-conscious or ashamed; you may worry about what the therapist thinks of you. Try to clear these thoughts out of your head and act like a consumer. The therapist is the one who's on the spot right now—not you. You should be polite, of course. But don't hesitate to probe thoroughly into the therapist's experience and credentials. Listen to the tone of his or her answers as well. Do you feel that this is a person you'll be able to trust? Do you feel comfortable with the voice and the attitude?

Unless you're in an emergency situation, it's important that you take the time to "shop wisely." You wouldn't hire a sitter for your child without talking with her first, and checking her references. Choosing a therapist is just the same. You may want to ask about his or her training, academic degrees, areas of specialization, professional affiliations, and licensure or certification. Edward Rydman asserts in *Finding the Right Counselor for You* that a good counselor will want you to have this information so that you will feel comfortable.

Beyond these basic questions about qualifications, you need to ask therapists about their approach. Do they have experience (and how much) treating postpartum women? How do they view difficulties in the postpartum period? What is their treatment philosophy? Do they try everything else before prescribing medication, or is medication their treatment of choice? You may want to keep shopping around if the therapist replies that depression or anxiety in the postpartum period is just like depression or anxiety at any other time. You may also want to avoid a therapist who does not see the postpartum period as an important life transition. The therapist should be able to give specific answers to your questions about postpartum psychological care. You may need to keep looking if the therapist seems to think of him/herself as an authority figure or expert whose orders you must obey, rather than as a facilitator or partner in your health care. Unless your choices are extremely limited, you can keep looking if a therapist makes you feel uncomfortable in any way.

During your initial conversation, you also need to ask questions about policies and costs. What does a session cost? How long does a session last? What is the cancellation policy? Can you make an appointment right now? Does the therapist offer an initial free consultation? Does the therapist ever include family members or significant others in the sessions? Can you bring the baby with you? What is the payment policy? You will also want to find out if your health insurance plan will cover any or all of your visits, and for medication if it's prescribed. If all of this is too overwhelming for you to do yourself, pass these instructions on to your partner or any other loving friend or family member. It's a bit like sending someone else out to buy your groceries—you'd better be specific about what you want, or you might wind up with a kitchen full of food you don't like.

Once you or your friends have found a therapist who comes highly recommended or who seems to be "speaking your language," you can schedule an initial evaluation or therapy session. You need to remember, at this point as well as throughout the therapy process, that you are in charge. As Dr. Rydman says in his book, the counseling session is for *you*. We recommend beginning the session by stating that you are looking for a therapist who will treat you as an equal, and see you as a partner. Such a therapist will want to hear your story, and will want you to take an active role in the session. Share what you have learned in this book about your difficulties, including your risk profile questionnaire from Chapter 3. Let the therapist know what you have tried, what has worked, and what has floundered. As you talk, pay attention to how the therapist communicates. Does he or she really seem to be listening? Do you understand his or her responses, or is it difficult to get past the jargon? Ask any questions that come up for you just as you did on the telephone. You'll want to decide at the end of the first session whether this is a person who can understand and be helpful to you. Trust your gut instincts. If you feel uncomfortable, unimportant, or misunderstood, you need to go elsewhere.

Counseling is a process, involving work over a period of time. You won't have all the answers by the end of the first session. But you're entitled, when this session is over, to feel that your therapist understands your situation, is empathetic and compassionate, and will be able to guide you in a positive direction. You deserve to have the sense that this person respects you and your personal values.

As professionals and women, we strongly believe that you are the consumer in this process, with all of a consumer's rights and prerogatives. You are paying for these sessions (or are paying for them through your insurance): you have an ultimate right to feel satisfied with the product. Be an educated consumer. Trust your judgment about what you need. Trust our judgment that what women need during a difficult postpartum adjustment is a health-care partner, one who can support and foster their own resources. Even though you're having problems now, you are ultimately in charge of your recovery.

We've spoken to many women who have had negative experiences with therapists who did not understand postpartum issues, or failed to see the importance of taking care of the immediate issues at hand. These therapists only made their patients feel worse. If the therapist you've selected wants to talk primarily about your early childhood, your parents, or your dreams—and if this doesn't feel right to you— you can feel perfectly justified in looking for help elsewhere. It's important to address the immediate concerns, like lack of sleep or panic attacks, before you deal with preexisting issues from your past. This here-and-now approach seems to work best for most postpartum women. Solve the daily concerns, and get to a more comfortable level of functioning, before you worry about underlying issues—unless, of course, you are seeing this as a time to finally tackle those underlying issues that have been plaguing you for years. In any case, be an educated consumer who knows she is entitled to get the help she needs. Therapists are as varied as all other people—some are smart, some are not so smart; some are likable, some are rather horrid. Ten different therapists may have ten different views about what is needed in a particular situation. Shop until you find one you feel you can work with. There should be some personal rapport on both sides; there should be mutual respect. Therapists are not always right, but it's essential that you find someone you can trust. You may need to interview several therapists before you find the right fit for you.

The Therapeutic Process

By the end of the initial session, you may have an idea about how this therapist views your situation, and what he or she would suggest as a treatment plan. In considering the therapist's outline of the help he or she plans to offer, it's important to place an emphasis on your own goals for your recovery. The treatment plan is open to negotiation between you and the therapist. It's appropriate to speak up right away about what parts of the plan you approve of, and what you might change. Nothing should be done during the course of your therapy that you don't feel completely comfortable doing. There's enough sense of losing control over one's life during the postpartum period without being bullied by your therapist into pursuing a course of treatment that feels wrong to you.

Even if you trust your therapist entirely, a leap of faith is sometimes required if you feel a bit worried about some aspects of the treatment plan. You may feel uncomfortable, for instance, about the idea of taking medication, even though your therapist feels that this would be the best and fastest way for you to recover. Your therapist may suggest a new behavior for you to try. Anything different from your usual habits may make you feel uncomfortable, simply because you haven't tried it before. It's important to sort out such feelings from any doubts you may have about the therapist's outlook or approach to therapy in general. Don't abandon a therapist you trust even if specific suggestions for treatment seem scary to you. You can and should have the opportunity to discuss your doubts and fears until you feel fully convinced that a given course is the best one.

June was a 19-year-old single mother who lived at home with her mother and younger brother. When her baby was six months old, June decided to talk to a therapist about the scary thoughts that had haunted her since her baby was born. June had daily worries that her baby might die of cancer. The baby's pediatrician reassured June that babies rarely contract any form of cancer. But it seemed that every time June opened the newspaper, or listened to the news on television, there was some report about devastating childhood illnesses. The thoughts played over and over again like a broken record in June's head: "Emily will get cancer, Emily will get cancer." Her mother advised June to stay busy, and just "not think about it." June went into a frenzy of housecleaning during her long days at home alone with the baby. But the thoughts wouldn't go away. June's grandmother, who lived next door, came over to keep her company, but that didn't help either.

June had no contact with Emily's father, who lived in another city, and had not spoken to her for months. She had no friends with children, and her friends from high school seemed so silly to her now. They talked about clothes, and going to clubs, and worried about what silly 19-year-old boys thought of them. June felt above this all. She had more important things on her mind, such as taking good care of her daughter and making a nice life for her. She hoped to get a job as soon as Emily was ready for pre-school, and maybe to go back to school herself. June's friends just couldn't relate to her concerns about the future, or her fears about Emily's health.

Even though June's mother was supporting her and the baby, and never complained about this, she'd lash out whenever June mentioned plans about eventually getting a job or moving away with Emily to a larger town where June might be able to enroll at a community college. June heard about Depression After Delivery on a daytime television program, called them, and got the name of a therapist.

In the initial session, June talked about the repetitive and scary thoughts that plagued her. Her idea was to learn more about this kind of thinking, and maybe to find a way to make it stop. She liked the therapist, who explained that the thoughts were due to biochemical changes in June's brain, along with the stress of all the new responsibility she faced now as a parent.

June found this information reassuring. The therapist suggested that they plan to work together for six sessions initially. During that time, the therapist would give June some specific tools to stop her scary thoughts. She also recommended that June contact a local support program for single parents. This could give June the opportunity to talk with other young people dealing with parenthood by themselves, and would provide comfort and an exchange of ideas.

Finally, the therapist suggested that June might want to take a look at where she was going with her life, and plan for her eventual independence from her mother. The stress of fighting with her mother every time she talked about making plans to leave home was probably adding to June's postpartum adjustment problems. The therapist wanted to know if June could bring her mother along for some family counseling sessions.

This idea completely terrified June. She felt that she'd never be able to talk about her plans for independence with her mother. Having her come to therapy would just make the fighting worse. June knew that her mother could be vindictive and mean, and was certain to pick on her at home for things that June said in the safety of the therapist's office. June expressed these fears to her therapist, even though she was afraid about the therapist getting mad at her, too, for speaking up. To her surprise, her therapist said that she understood June's reluctance. They could postpone that part of the treatment plan until later, and evaluate it then.

After several weeks, June found that the therapist's techniques for stopping the disaster thoughts about Emily were working. June wrote her thoughts down in a notebook when she had them, and put the notebook away in her dresser drawer. She also wore a rubber band on her wrist that she snapped every time one of the obsessive thoughts about Emily's health entered her head. She was actually feeling much better. Whole days went by when she didn't have any scary thoughts at all.

But the fighting with her mother was getting worse, and June found herself talking about that more frequently during her therapy sessions. When her therapist again raised the idea of family sessions, June was not as upset this time. Sure, talking with her mother would be difficult and she might snipe at June once they got home. But her mother seemed to be angry at her much of the time, anyway—June reasoned that maybe it would help, after all, to get a third party involved. She had come to trust her therapist, and felt she could take that leap of faith.

Before June invited her mother to attend a session with her she and the therapist carefully planned her strategy for discussing the independence issue without raising her mother's hackles. They also laid out some ground rules for the sessions. The main rule was that neither June nor her mother could bring up the sessions in an angry or otherwise negative way when they were at home. This made June feel somewhat protected, especially when her mother agreed to abide by the rules. After a couple of family sessions, June and her mother found that talking things out made their life together much smoother. June started a first-year college correspondence course to give her a jump-start on her education once she and Emily were ready to move to a bigger town.

Your therapist should respect your treatment goals and your sense of an appropriate time frame for your recovery. If your therapist believes that your goals are unrealistic within that time frame, or if some of his or her suggestions sound scary to you, you can work together to modify the treatment plan. Scary ideas can be put on the back burner for a while. Or you can agree to try things in modified form, or in small doses. Your treatment plan is not cast in stone, but should be flexible, based on what you feel as you move through the process of your recovery. You may feel most comfortable committing to a small number of sessions at first, such as three or four. You'll know the therapist's working style by then, and will have a sense about whether you are getting what you need. Your treatment plan may include individual sessions, group sessions, and couple or family sessions, depending on what you and your therapist feel would be most helpful. Above all, your treatment plan should focus your efforts on the problems that seem biggest to you right now. Remember—you're the consumer here; you're paying for a service. If you're not working on the issues that are most important to you, you have a right to make your wishes known and get your therapy back on track (or switch therapists).

"Talking" Therapy

You may wonder how counseling actually works. What is it about talking things out that can make you feel better? Maybe you feel as if you've already talked about your postpartum issues until you're blue in the face. What good can more talking do?

There are several differences between talking things out with a friend and talking them out with a mental health professional. First of all, the counselor is trained to get you to look at your issues in new ways and from a broader perspective. A good counselor is a facilitator, who will listen without judging or punishing you. As Dr. Rydman writes in his book, counseling requires you to be an active participant—your therapist can't "fix" you without your participation any more than your parents could have taught you to ride a bike if you only stood by the sidelines and watched.

Therapy may help you discover a different way to tackle a parenting issue, master a new self-care skill, or broaden your expectations of your

Types of Therapy

Individual therapy. In individual therapy, the emphasis is usually on the individual person's thoughts, actions, and feelings. Discussion will usually center on what the individual can do differently. Individual therapy is needed when most of the client's concerns do not seem focused on the partner or family relationships.

Conjoint therapy. Conjoint therapy involves more than one person—a couple, an entire family, an adult and a child, an adult and the adult's parents, and so on. This is also called marital or family therapy. In this type of therapy, the focus is usually on the interaction between the parties involved. Discussion might center around improving their interactions or communication. Conjoint therapy is usually needed when the problems are in the relationship rather than in one individual.

Group therapy. In group therapy, several people meet with one or more therapists to discuss similar problems. Problems may be closely related, with all participants being in the same life situation. Or the focus may be broader, such as in groups that focus on women's issues in general or mixed (men's and women's) groups with a focus on relationship difficulties.

Cognitive therapy. In cognitive therapy, the focus is mainly on how the client thinks and views the world. The therapist may adopt an active, teaching focus, helping the client spot maladaptive thinking patterns and replace them with more effective patterns. Emphasis is on the present.

Behavior therapy. In behavior therapy, the therapist focuses primarily on how a person acts, rather than on underlying thoughts or emotions. The therapist and client work as a team to replace negative behaviors with more positive ones. The emphasis is on actually doing things differently in the present, with little attention paid to past events.

Systems therapy. In systems therapy, emphasis is placed on the relationships (systems) in which the client is involved. In most variations of systems therapy, the therapist focuses on changing the habitual patterns of interaction between the individuals rather than on changing the individuals themselves. Attention is paid to how the family members were shaped by the families in which they were raised, and how those influences continue in the present day. This therapy is fairly action-oriented, with focus on developing more adaptive ways to relate to others.

Psychodynamic/analytic therapy. In psychodynamic therapy, or analysis, focus is on a client's underlying, unconscious motivations or urges. The goal is for a client to understand, or gain insight into, these previously unconscious issues. Psychodynamic therapists usually take a much less active role, allowing the client to take the lead. Sometimes they may listen without responding at all. The focus is more on past events, dreams, and early childhood than it is in any of the other types of therapy described here.

Interpersonal therapy. Interpersonal therapy stresses the importance of positive relationships to well-being. The therapist and client work together to evaluate the effectiveness of the client's current relationships, and on helping the client develop relationship skills. Focus is on the here-and-now, rather than on the past.

Feminist therapy. Feminist therapy is not based on politics, but rather on the idea that women may be more prone to depression from living in a culture in which sexism, discrimination, and violence against women are prevalent. Understanding these cultural influences is seen as essential, but the goal of therapy is not to place blame or provide excuses. Once this understanding is achieved, feminist therapy encourages women to value themselves as people, to increase the awareness of their own power, and become active in building better lives for themselves. The therapist serves as a guide and support.

Eclectic therapy. Eclectic therapists use techniques from more than one of the types of therapy listed here, adapting what works for individual clients. The approach described in the self-care section of this book is eclectic, borrowing from cognitive-behavioral, systems, feminist, and interpersonal therapy. Our approach is action-oriented, based in the present, and aimed at empowering women.

new role. What you say in your sessions is strictly confidential, within certain legal limits; and so you may be more open and honest than you would be with a friend or family member. (Since these limits vary from state to state, you need to discuss this issue with your therapist.) In that counseling requires that you look at negative feelings and problems within your postpartum adjustment, it can definitely feel painful; and it's usually very hard work. It can also be stressful, which may feel particularly unappealing to you right now when you have so much stress in your life already. Talking therapy requires self-examination and you may not always like what you see. It can be hard to admit, even to yourself, that you doubt your skills as a parent or your decision to have a baby. And yet having the help and suggestions of a nonjudgmental, supportive expert in postpartum adjustment problems can give you the optimism you need to feel that your life can improve, and your problems can be worked out. Just believing in your power to make things better can give you the strength and determination to go on.

You're highly unlikely to get all the answers you're looking for in just one counseling session. Therapy takes time. When you've mastered the tools you need to cope with your postpartum changes, and when your life feels manageable again, you'll be ready to end your therapy. Termination is part of the therapeutic process. You may have mixed feelings about it. It may feel scary; you may worry that no one will ever listen to you so closely and kindly again. You may also be relieved to finally feel so much better, and to have achieved the postpartum picture you'd envisioned before the birth. Ending therapy may feel like a sort of graduation.

Your therapist will talk with you about how to maintain the changes you've achieved. He or she may help you devise a checklist of warning signs to watch for, to avoid losing the gains you've made, and to enable you to stay on track.

Before you embark on the counseling process, you need to realize that there are limitations as well to what therapy can do for you. Sometimes people end up feeling dissatisfied with their therapy or therapist because they expected too much. Their goals may be unrealistic. Their feelings from the past may be too strong to deal with in a short period of time. You may need to work on your own with what you have learned in therapy for several months, or longer; maybe even for the rest of your life. That's why a good therapist doesn't "solve" your problems, but gives you tools so that you can learn to cope on your own as you face the other stresses and difficult transitions that life deals out.

If you feel disappointed about the limitations of your therapist or the therapy itself, you can discuss these issues during your counseling sessions. A competent, supportive therapist will not be afraid to look at his or her role in your disappointment. It's important for you to gauge your own expectations as well. Were they realistic? Did the therapist promise you something that wasn't delivered? Do *you* feel that the time has arrived to end your therapy, or do you need the continuing support? If so, make your needs and feelings known. As the consumer in this process, you are entitled to end therapy when *you* want to.

One other note. It can feel painful after opening your heart so completely to your therapist, and feeling so well understood, to suddenly face life without this staunch advocate and friend. And yet, therapists and friends are very different—not only in the way they listen, but in the function they serve. With few exceptions, a therapist will not "continue to be your friend" after therapy ends. This is not because therapists are friendly only when you're paying an hourly rate, but because of a professional code which makes it important for the therapist to remain available in a therapeutic role if you ever need help again. A therapist who crosses the line and becomes your friend can never again have that special distance that allows the therapeutic process to happen. If you feel sad saying goodbye—and many people do—you can comfort yourself with the thought that your wise counselor will always be there for you, waiting to help, if you're in need.

Sometimes, talk therapy alone is insufficient to tackle a woman's postpartum adjustment problems. Psychoactive medications such as anti-anxiety or antidepressant drugs, may be needed to bring your body and mind back into balance.

This is certainly not true for every woman. But if you wish to explore the question of whether such medications might aid your recovery, continue reading the rest of this chapter.

Medications in the Postpartum Period

Psychoactive, or psychiatric medication can be beneficial for some women in the postpartum period, although it should only be chosen as an alternative after very careful consideration. These medications include several categories of drugs that may relieve symptoms commonly experienced by women with postpartum emotional reactions. These categories of drugs are

- Antidepressants
- Anti-anxiety medications
- Antimania medications
- Antipsychotic drugs
- Sleep medications

Hormone therapy is also sometimes used to treat postpartum emotional reactions. These various interventions will be described in the rest of this chapter, with general guidelines about when they should be considered.

You may be wondering why medication would be helpful at all during a postpartum emotional reaction. In Chapter 3 we talked about the issue of psychological versus biochemical causes of postpartum reactions. We believe that postpartum adjustment problems are caused by a combination of factors, psychological and emotional as well as hormonal and biological. Psychiatric medications can be extremely helpful in enabling postpartum women to feel better faster, particularly when biochemical stresses have "tipped the balance." These drugs influence your biochemical balance, restoring your brain chemicals, or brain hormones, to their previous state. Treatment with these medications can work immediately, or can take days or weeks before a change is noticed. The effect may be lasting, or may disappear as soon as the medication wears off. The period of time you would need to stay on the drug varies from medication to medication.

We cannot stress emphatically enough that breastfeeding is not compatible with many medications, including most psychoactive drugs. If you are committed to breastfeeding your baby, you may want to consider all other alternatives before resorting to medication—because taking these drugs in many cases will mean that you'll have to wean your baby. There is an unfortunate tendency in much of the medical community now to see postpartum reactions as primarily biochemical, and so easily and quickly "fixed" by psychoactive medication.

We do not feel that these drugs should be considered as such an easy answer, particularly if taking them means that you have to wean your baby. There are certainly other means to try before you try psychoactive drugs. These alternative methods include self-care and psychotherapy, which are described in Chapter 4 and the first part of this chapter.

Breastfeeding is important for nutritional and for psychological reasons, for the baby and for the mother, and for the relationship between the two. Medication is critical for some women in speeding their postpartum emotional recovery. But that fact needs to be balanced carefully against the importance of breastfeeding.

There is recent research which suggests that mothers may be able to take some psychoactive medications while continuing to breastfeed their babies. The most up-to-date information we've been able to gather on this subject is provided later in this chapter. Your decision about whether to take medication, and possibly wean your baby earlier than you had planned, should not be hastily or carelessly considered. You have to decide what is right for you and your baby. You need to get as many facts as you can. With the help of your partner and health-care professionals, weigh the pros and cons of taking the medication and weaning earlier than you'd planned. Don't put yourself in the position of having to abandon breastfeeding if that doesn't seem like the best alternative to you. You should take medication only if it appears to be the sole route to recovery you haven't yet tried, or if you're in a life-and-death situation in which medication seems to be the only answer (such as if you're suicidal).

When should you explore the use of psychoactive drugs? If you're working diligently on a self-care plan, as outlined in this book, and still don't feel better within two to three weeks, you may want to explore medication as an alternative. If you're committed to breastfeeding your baby, you will want to try psychotherapy before medication, except in the most extreme cases, as described above.

Symptoms Readily Affected by Medication

- Sleep disturbances

- Fatigue

- Restlessness, agitation

- Panic attacks

- Lack of ability to feel pleasure in anything

- Mood variations throughout the day (feeling worse in the morning especially)

- Appetite changes

- Decreased sex drive

- Obsessive thoughts

- Psychotic symptoms

- Concentration difficulties and forgetfulness

Adapted and used with permission of publisher from *Clinical Psychopharmocology Made Ridiculously Simple* by John Preston and James Johnson. Miami: MedMaster, Inc., 1993.

There are certain symptoms that seem to respond especially well to medication. These categories of symptoms are summarized in the chart above. Many of these symptoms can be associated in some cases with an underlying biochemical imbalance, which accounts for their responsiveness to medication.

Many women find medication to be a useful adjunct to psychotherapy and self-care. Sometimes the physical symptoms of depression, agitation, panic, or sleep disturbance can be so strong that you can't focus on your self-care plan, even with the help of a therapist. Turning to medication does not mean that you are giving up on your previous efforts, or that your previous efforts have failed. You are not becoming a drug addict, nor are you relying on the medication to medically "fix" everything for you. But in some cases, medication can lift the fog that prevents you from doing what you need to do to take care of yourself. It's not a magic bullet, it doesn't simply make everything better. What it can do is give you enough symptom relief so that you can actually use the resources you have to help yourself. Instead of being overwhelmed with fatigue, or caught up in obsessive thoughts, you can begin to think things through again, or you can learn to see things in a new light. Medication can help some people "see the forest through the trees." When you can calm down, or get some rest, or see the bright side of your world again, you can get on with the business of your recovery. In such cases, medication can be a real lifesaver.

When Your Therapist Recommends Medication

Perhaps you are actively working on your self-care plan. You may be working in psychotherapy with a counselor you are coming to trust. It can come as a surprise if your therapist suggests that you would benefit from medication.

Does this mean that the therapist doesn't believe that talking therapy is helping you? Not necessarily. You should discuss this issue with your therapist. Why does he or she believe that medication would be helpful? What symptoms or behaviors is the therapist using as criteria for choosing medication?

Many therapists—especially psychiatrists—may view postpartum emotional reactions as being primarily biological in nature. These helping professionals are likely to recommend or prescribe psychoactive medication fairly often. Many other therapists view postpartum emotional difficulties as being largely due to psychological, or life stress, causes. Knowing where your therapist stands on this issue can help you evaluate his or her recommendation that you begin to take medication for symptom relief. If you are committed to breastfeeding, be sure and ask what other options are available for treatment besides the medication in question. You have a right to question any course of treatment, and to find a different helper if your questions aren't satisfactorily answered.

Psychoactive medications can only be prescribed by medical doctors. Psychologists, social workers, and other types of counselors can only offer psychotherapy. If your therapist is not an M.D. or D.O., he or she will have to work in consultation with a psychiatrist or another medical doctor who can prescribe medication if you choose that option. In addition to psychiatrists, many family practitioners, obstetrician/gynecologists, internists, and general practitioners may prescribe psychoactive drugs. If a therapist recommends that you take these medications, but can't arrange for you to obtain them, feel free to ask about what other options are available to you. You and your therapist can probably work out a plan for obtaining a prescription from an appropriate source.

Before you take any medication, however, you will want to evaluate any other possible sources for your symptoms. How is your health overall? Have you ruled out other physical causes for your symptoms? Are you taking any other medications that could be causing you to feel this way? Many medications can cause depression, anxiety, and sleep problems. As you think about the answers to these questions, be sure to include nonprescription drugs in your consideration. Do you drink a great deal of coffee, tea, or cola, or do you eat chocolate? Caffeine can cause agitation. Do you smoke cigarettes? You shouldn't overlook the effects of nicotine. Is your diet overloaded with processed sugar? Low blood sugar can be a culprit in mood swings. Do you drink alcoholic beverages every night in an effort to relax? Alcohol close to bedtime can actually cause increased insomnia. Regularly prescribed medications, such as antihypertensives (for high blood pressure), corticosteriods, hormones in birth control pills or other medications, antiparkinson drugs, and anti-anxiety drugs can all cause depression. Amphetamines, asthma medications, caffeine, withdrawal from tranquilizers, cocaine, nasal decongestant sprays, and steroids can all cause anxiety. After you've looked at your use of other drugs, be sure to inform your health-care practitioner of any medications you are taking and ask about how these might react with any psychiatric drug under consideration.

You may think that taking psychoactive medication will make you feel better almost instantly. Once again, our old friend "expectations" is at work. Prepare yourself not to be disappointed if medications don't work for you. Drugs are not the answer for every new mother by any means. They do not remove the need to make changes in your life. They often take several weeks before they create noticeable changes in your mood. And "shopping" for the most helpful medication can be as involved a process as shopping for a therapist or selecting a babysitter. You may not find the one drug that works for you on the first try. Side effects may be unbearable, outweighing any positive effects of the drug. You may need to take more than one drug in combination. It's not uncommon for a combination of antidepressants and anti-anxiety agents to be the best treatment for postpartum symptoms. What works for another woman in your support group may not work for you. Life circumstances and body chemistry are different for every woman. Experiment as needed, with your doctor's support and guidance. And have hope that you will find something that is right for you.

When Drugs Are the Only Choice

There are several postpartum reactions for which medication is absolutely required. The first of these is postpartum psychosis. When a person acts psychotic, there is a definite biochemical basis for their symptoms, and medication is the required treatment. It's crucial not to delay if a woman is exhibiting psychotic symptoms—if she's having hallucinations, hearing voices, or is otherwise out of touch with reality—for there is a clear risk to the woman and her infant if proper treatment is not given.

Likewise, postpartum mania requires medication. Again, there is a biological basis for mania, whose symptoms include extreme agitation, seemingly boundless energy despite little or no sleep, and the inability to follow one task through to completion before turning to another project. If left untreated, mania can quickly escalate into psychosis.

If someone you know is experiencing any psychotic or manic symptoms (as described in Chapter 2), help them to get immediate medical attention.

Antidepressants

Antidepressants are the most frequently prescribed medications for women with postpartum emotional reactions. Antidepressants fall into two main categories: 1) tricyclics and tricycliclike compounds and 2) MAO inhibitors.

Researchers who study depression believe that depressive symptoms are caused by an imbalance of certain brain chemicals, called neurotransmitters. The neurotransmitters more often identified as influencing depression are norepinephrine and serotonin. Antidepressant medications work by restoring the balance of these chemicals in the brain. In other words, these drugs work by retraining the brain to be more sensitive to these natural chemicals, and to manufacture more of them.

Different medications seem to affect brain chemicals in distinct ways. Some medications appear to affect some symptoms more than others. Your health-care professional should take these differences into account when deciding what drug might work best for you.

Researchers across the country who are studying postpartum women are finding that about half of the women seem to respond more to the related tricycliclike compounds, called selective serotonergic reuptaker inhibitors. See the chart that follows for the generic and brand names of these drugs, listed by categories.

MAO inhibitors have not been widely used or studied with postpartum women. This is because these drugs can cause dangerous reactions when taken in conjunction with certain foods. Individuals who take these drugs must greatly restrict their diets to avoid negative reactions. Nevertheless, research *is* being done with MAO inhibitors, and the future may show them to be extremely effective with postpartum women. The question is still open.

If you are planning to take antidepressants, there are some key points to remember. First of all, these drugs generally do not begin to work for 10-21 days. You'll have to take the prescribed medication for this long before you notice any improvement in your symptoms. Secondly, these drugs are not "happy pills." The symptoms that most often respond to treatment with antidepressants are the physiological ones. You may find that you are beginning to sleep better, are less tired, are less easily irritated, or are crying less.

You also need to realize that you may have side effects, such as dry mouth or nausea. Have your physician or pharmacist explain these side effects completely: you can also read about them in the *Physicians Desk Reference*, a book that is available at every doctor's office, pharmacy, and reference library. Many side effects pass within several days or a week. Adjusting the dose or the time of day at which you take the medication can help minimize unpleasant side effects.

Antidepressant Medications

Tricyclics

Generic Name	Brand Name	Usual Daily Dosage	Key Effect
Imiprimine	*Tofranil*	150-300 mg	S>N
Desiprimine	*Norpramin*	150-300 mg	N
Amitryptiline	*Elavil*	150-300 mg	S
Notriptyline	*Aventyl, Pamelor*	75-125 mg	N>S
Protriptyline	*Vivactil*	15-40 mg	N
Trimiprimine	*Surmontil*	100-300 mg	S
Doxepin	*Sinequan, Adapin*	150-300 mg	S
Maprotiline	*Ludiomil*	150-225 mg	N
Amoxapine	*Asendin*	150-400 mg	N
Trazodone	*Desyrel*	150-400 mg	S
Bupropion	*Wellbutrin*	200-450 mg	*
Venlafaxine	*Effexor*	75-375 mg	S, N

Selective Serotonergic Reuptake Inhibitors

Fluoxetine	*Prozac*	20-80 mg	S
Sertraline	*Zoloft*	50-200 mg	S
Paroxetine	*Paxil*	20-60 mg	S
Clomipramine	*Anafranil*	150-300 mg	S

MAO Inhibitors

Phenelzine	*Nardil*	30-90 mg	E, N, S
Tranylcypromine	*Parnate*	20-60 mg	E, N, S
Isocarboxazid	*Marplan*	20-40 mg	E, N, S

E = epinephrine is the primary chemical affected
N = norepinephrine is the primary chemical affected
S = serotonin is the primary chemical affected
* = main chemical affected is uncertain—may be dopamine

Adapted and used with permission from *Handbook of Clinical Psychopharmacology for Therapists* by John D. Preston, John O'Neal, and Mary Talaga. Oakland, CA: New Harbinger Publications, 1994.

How long you will need to take the medication varies from person to person. You are less likely to relapse, falling back into the full force of the symptoms, if you stay on the medication for four to six months after you notice that your symptoms are gone. If you quit taking the medication sooner than this, you may be severely disappointed to find that your symptoms reappear. When you've been on the medication as long as you and your health-care provider feel is adequate, you can begin to decrease the dose gradually. It's usually important to achieve stability for a month to six weeks after each time you lower the dosage before reducing the dosage even further.

Don't drink alcoholic beverages while taking these medications. Alcohol can interfere with its positive effects.

Finally, you need to reassure yourself and others around you that antidepressant medication is not addictive. When the chemical balance in your brain is restored, you will no longer need the medication.

What if the medication does not seem to be working? Most often, this is because the dosage is too low. Your health-care provider will probably raise the dose if you notice no effects within 10-21 days. If, however, you have been on a high dose for 3-4 weeks and feel no better, it may be that this drug will not work for you. Frequently, physicians will add a low dose of lithium, which is a drug either used alone or to boost the effect of antidepressants. If you still have no response, it's probably time to switch to another medication.

As described above, some drugs seem to work best on the brain chemical norepinephrine, while others affect the serotonin. If the first drug you tried acted primarily on the norepinephrine, you may then want to try a drug which will balance the serotonin. It's still sort of a crapshoot, as researchers haven't matched these chemical reactions to specific symptoms. If you still do not have success, the choice may be to try an MAO inhibitor.

Some women will find that antidepressant medication, however many different drugs they try, is just not successful. In some rare cases, electroconvulsive therapy—also known as ECT or "shock therapy"—has been shown to be extremely effective. It's a very costly procedure, because hospitalization and highly trained personnel are required for its administration. It generally has been given a bad rap because of its frequent misuse in the past; as a result, psychiatrists are not routinely trained in ECT, making it not readily available. If a facility and physician you know of possess considerable experience with ECT, it is a perfectly safe treatment alternative. Postpartum women who undergo ECT often find that they have a relatively quick and gratifying recovery.

Anti-Anxiety Medications

Anti-anxiety medications are also known as minor tranquilizers, anxiolytics, and benzodiazepines. Use of specific medications to treat anxiety depends a great deal on the exact symptoms that plague you.

Anti-Anxiety Medications

Generic Name	Brand Name	Usual Dosage	Used to Treat
Alprazolam	*Xanax*	5-40 mg	Stress, panic
Clonazepam	*Klonopin*	.5-4 mg	Stress, panic
Prazepam	*Centrax*	20-60 mg	Stress
Lorazepam	*Ativan*	2-6 mg	Stress
Clorazepate	*Tranxene*	15-60 mg	Stress
Oxazepam	*Serax*	30-120 mg	Stress
Chlordiaze-poxide	*Librium*	15-100 mg	Stress
Diazepam	*Valium*	5-40 mg	Stress
Buspirone	*BuSpar*	5-40 mg	Generalized anxiety

Stress = anxiety related to a specific stressor (also called a "situational anxiety")
Panic = panic disorder—i.e., repeated panic attacks
Generalized anxiety = anxiety that invades most aspects of one's life

Adapted and used with permission from *Handbook of Clinical Psychopharmacology for Therapists* by John D. Preston, John O'Neal, and Mary Talaga. Oakland, CA: New Harbinger Publications, 1994.

For instance, a physician might prescribe one medication for panic attacks, and a different medication for stress-related anxiety. It's important to explain your symptoms precisely, and in as much detail as possible, so that your doctor can prescribe an anti-anxiety drug that has been shown to be helpful for each symptom. The chart on the next page shows the usual dosage and use for nine anti-anxiety medications.

Medication for Panic Attacks

Many postpartum women describe panic attacks that last only a matter of minutes. If you have anxiety that seems to continue for hours or days, this would be characterized as a more general anxiety, probably related to specific stressors, such as taking the baby out in public. Your anxiety may be much broader based—a general anxiety about your life now—seemingly unconnected to anything specific. It's also possible to have panic attacks on top of a more general feeling of anxiety. Look in

Chapter 2 at the descriptions of the different types of anxiety experienced by postpartum women. Pinpointing your symptoms can be extremely important in helping your physician decide on the best medication for you.

If you have had true panic attacks, which come out of the blue and then quickly subside, you may find that you have also developed what is called anticipatory anxiety as a result. With anticipatory anxiety, you may find that you have begun to avoid situations where more panic attacks may occur. You avoid being alone, for example, if your previous panic attacks happened when you were alone. This avoidance may soon become a habit, which also needs treatment. Therapy for panic attacks, therefore, usually requires two phases. In the first phase, you treat the panic; when this is more under control, you then address the habit of avoidance.

In the first phase of this therapy, the goal is to eliminate or decrease the frequency and strength of your panic attacks. This is often accomplished with either benzodiazepines, such as aprazolam (*Xanax*), or antidepressants (tricyclics or MAO inhibitors). While the benzodiazepines may act very quickly, you may develop a tolerance to them—so that they'll stop working—if you use them for an extended period of time. This risk needs to be considered in prescribing them.

If antidepressants are used, there is no such risk. They work more slowly, however, than the benzodiazepines. Often, physicians will prescribe benzodiazepines for use during the two or three weeks while you are waiting for the antidepressants to take effect.

Once you are having fewer and/or milder panic attacks, you can begin to tackle the anticipatory anxiety described above. This is best done by slowly returning to those situations that worry you: psychologists call this *systematic desensitization*. In gradual steps, you go back into the situation in which you had a panic attack, in order to learn that you can handle it without panicking. As you discover that you can cope with that situation successfully, your need to worry about it in advance will decrease. It's important to tackle this process slowly, and with a lot of help and understanding from family, friends, and your medical support team.

On two different occasions, Patti had a panic attack while bathing her baby, both times while her husband was at work. Fearing that it would happen again, Patti refused to bathe the baby, and her husband took over the task for several weeks. Patti's fear escalated to the point where she was afraid of being alone with the baby. So she was not only feeling like she couldn't care for her baby, but she also cried every morning when her husband left for work. Some days she cried all day long.

After seven days of crying, Patti called her childbirth educator and was given the name of a psychiatrist specializing in panic attacks. Patti made an immediate appointment. Her husband accompanied her, caring for the baby during the session. The physician prescribed an antidepressant and a benzodiazepine for the panic. She took the benzodiazepine just when she felt her anxiety beginning to build—just before bathtime—while she took the antidepressant every evening at bedtime. Patti began to feel better within two weeks. She was crying less, and was more tolerant of staying alone while her husband went to work. But she still couldn't bring herself to give the baby a bath. When Patti checked in with her doctor, they worked on a plan to slowly increase her confidence about bathing the baby. On the first night of putting the plan into effect, she watched from the doorway while her husband bathed the baby. Seeing that she could keep fairly calm while watching, the next night she came into the bathroom to watch the bath. Patti gradually took on some of the responsibility for the bath, beginning with just washing the baby's feet and working her way up. When she could wash the baby completely on her own, her husband gradually inched his way out of the bathroom, standing farther away from Patti each night, until he was out of sight and earshot. In this step-by-step manner, Patti was once again able to give the baby a bath on her own without fear of having a panic attack. She worked with her doctor to decrease her medication progressively as well. First she cut her dose of the anti-anxiety medication. She stayed on the antidepressant for about eight months more, and then slowly tapered off on that drug as well.

Medication for Situational Anxiety

If your anxiety seems to focus primarily on certain stresses, your physician will likely prescribe medication to be taken at those stressful times. Benzodiazepines—which is the medication Patti took in conjunction with an antidepressant—can also be taken on an as-needed basis when you begin to feel anxious; they generally help the anxiety subside fairly rapidly. Benzodiazepines are mainly taken for short periods of time for stress-related anxiety. These drugs have a common side effect of sleepiness which may be extremely helpful if you're also having difficulty sleeping. But it can be difficult to balance the need to decrease your anxiety against a concern about becoming overly sedated.

Another possible problem with using benzodiazepines to treat anxiety is that they may cause a euphoric "rush" when the medication enters the bloodstream. This euphoria can be addictive for people who are prone to reliance on drugs. If you have a history of addictive behavior—with drugs, food, or exercise—it's critical that you inform your physician of this if he or she is talking about prescribing a benzodiazepine for you. The goal of using medication is to minimize your present difficulties, not to add new problems or revive old difficulties.

Ginger was a 24-year-old first-time mother with a healthy baby boy. Ginger's mother came to help out from day one, when Ginger and her husband Lee brought their baby home from the hospital. All went well the first several days, until Ginger and her mother bundled the baby into his car seat and headed off to the pediatrician's office for a bilirubin check

(Lee had noticed that the baby's skin looked slightly yellow). On the way there, they were waiting at a stoplight on a one-way street when a pick-up truck came around the corner too fast just as a taxi pulled out from the curb. The truck skidded and rammed into the driver's side rear door. Ginger's mother had been driving, with Ginger sitting behind her to watch the baby in his car seat, which was in the middle of the backseat. The truck driver stopped, and police and ambulance were called. Ginger and her mother were shaken, but unharmed, and the baby was fine. He wakened from his dozing, and screamed for several minutes until Ginger got him out of the car seat, and patted and rocked him in her arms. The car door was so damaged that it could not be opened. Ginger, her mother, and the baby were checked by paramedics, and taken on to the pediatrician's office for further checking.

Lee met his family at the doctor's office, where everyone proved to be physically fine. Lee drove them all home. On the ride, Ginger could barely contain her anxiety. She decided to avoid riding in the car for several days, hoping that a break would help her overcome her anxiety. When she even thought about getting into the car, she began to feel anxious, envisioning the accident again. She knew her anxiety didn't make sense, because she had never once been in an accident before this one, and odds were against another one occurring in the next week or so. Ginger tried to talk herself out of her fear. She even tried going for rides to force herself to overcome it, but felt extremely anxious and uncomfortable. When her mother's visit was about to come to an end, ten days later, Ginger and Lee decided that they'd better do something that would allow Ginger to drive again. Her mother had been doing all the necessary errands, but Ginger was about to have to take over that task.

Ginger called her obstetrician, who recommended that she take *Xanax* for a week or two when preparing to get in the car. For the final three days of her mother's visit, Ginger took the medication whenever they needed to go somewhere, but she still let her mother drive. Finally feeling somewhat more confident, Ginger drove her mother to the airport. The medication gave back her sense of being in control; she only took it for two more days after her mother left. The *Xanax* helped Ginger overcome her fear enough so that she could tackle driving again.

Medication for Generalized Anxiety

For more general, overwhelming anxiety, physicians often prescribe buspirone. Sold under the brand name *BuSpar*, this drug is much slower to act than *Xanax*. It may take two to four weeks before you feel some positive effect and it must be taken every day. If you find that you feel anxious about nearly everything, buspirone may be helpful for you. It does not, however, seem to be effective as a way to manage panic attacks.

Abigail was a 31-year-old single mother who gave birth to twins. She worked as a teacher, and planned to take only a four-week leave before she returned to her classroom. Money was tight, and Abigail worried a great deal about how she would manage financially. How could she pay for two tiny babies in day care, let alone provide everything she wanted for her children's lives? She became overcome with anxiety whenever she even thought about the future. Abigail found a kind neighbor who ran a home day-care center that accepted newborns. Abigail trusted this woman, and decided to enroll the twins there when she returned to work.

But things didn't go smoothly for Abigail. She spent at least an hour each day with stomache cramps, lying on a couch in the teacher's lounge, while an office aide covered her classes. Then Abigail began to break out in a strange rash. Her hands and arms and neck itched, which affected her concentration at work. When she was home with the babies, she felt okay so long as she avoided the news on TV or any mention of "financial security" in TV commercials. Abigail had great difficulty sleeping, even though she was exhausted. She frequently woke in a sweat from a bad dream which she could not recall.

After about three weeks of this misery, Abigail decided to see her family doctor about the rash and stomach pains. She had tried over-the-counter creams and lotions for her skin, and was tired of chewing antacid tablets. The doctor examined her thoroughly, and gently explained that he thought her ailments were due to her intense worries. He prescribed *BuSpar*, less stress, and a single-parent support group at a local Y.

Abigail took the medication and attended the support group. Through the group, she became acquainted with another single mother who was running a home day-care center so that she could stay at home with her own three-year-old son. This woman offered to care for Abigail's twins for considerably less money than she'd been paying to her neighbor. After Abigail switched day-care situations, she began to make changes in her evening schedule as well, allowing the babies to lie on a blanket on the floor while she actually sat down and ate a meal, rather than trying to juggle one baby on her shoulder and the other on her knee while she grabbed a bite of bread or a drink of juice. She also made an effort to meet socially one night a week with several other new moms. As she got to know these women, she began to feel comfortable trading babysitting with them so that each of them could have some evening time off. She continued to take her medication, and tried to reduce the level of stress in her life. By the time six weeks had passed, Abigail found that she hadn't had a nightmare or stomach pain for three weeks running; and her rash had cleared up completely.

Medication for Postpartum Obsessive-Compulsive Disorder

Obsessive-compulsive thoughts are another anxiety reaction which responds readily to psychoactive medication. Many women find that the antidepressants that influence the brain chemical serotonin—particularly

Anafranil, Prozac, Zoloft, and *Paxil*—are effective in eliminating obsessive thoughts. Sometimes physicians prescribe an anti-anxiety agent, such as *Xanax* or *Klonipin*, to decrease anxiety about the thoughts while waiting for the antidepressant to take effect. The anti-anxiety medication (benzodiazepine) can then be gradually decreased over time, allowing the antidepressant to take over.

Libby was a 19-year-old mother, married only two weeks before she became pregnant with her daughter. When the baby was three days old, Libby began to have disturbing thoughts about harming her. What if she just put the baby in the microwave? What if she dropped the baby on the steps? These thoughts seemed to come out of nowhere. Libby was puzzled, and talked about the thoughts with her husband. He reacted in a supportive manner, telling her he was sure it was nothing to worry about. She hadn't done it, had she? Libby's husband worked in a local hospital kitchen as a chef-in-training. The next day, he pulled aside one of the nurses he had come to know slightly, and told her about his wife's concern. The nurse brought him a magazine article on postpartum obsessive-compulsive reaction, which explained the biochemical cause of the thoughts that Libby was having. When Libby read this, she felt much relieved. She called the hospital where the baby had been born, and learned that they had a community mental health clinic she'd be able to visit. She went the next day, and as she wasn't breastfeeding, she started on the antidepressant *Anafranil* right away. Within two weeks, the thoughts had disappeared entirely.

Antipsychotic Medications

When a new mother is having psychotic symptoms, she requires antipsychotic medication. This medication can restore chemical balance in the brain, relieving the symptoms of hallucinations, delusions, and confusion quite rapidly. Because many antipsychotic medications have negative side effects, they are generally started at low doses, with the dosage increased as necessary. These side effects range from drowsiness, dry mouth, constipation, urinary retention, and dizziness to muscular rigidity, tremors, muscle spasms, and slowed motor responses. Additional medications—called anticholinergic agents—are often given to control these side effects. Your physician must find the correct balance of medications that will eliminate the psychotic symptoms without overwhelming you with side effects. Once the symptoms are controlled, remaining on the medication may be necessary for up to one year. If the psychotic episode is not the first you've had, it may be necessary to take the medication for an even longer period of time. Some common antipsychotic medications are listed in the chart that follows.

Melissa had her first baby when she was 35. The birth and hospital stay went well, and Melissa and the baby went home within 36 hours.

Antipsychotic Medications

Generic Name	Brand Name	Usual Daily Dosage
Chlorpromazine	Thorazine	50-1500 mg
Thioridazine	Mellaril	150-800 mg
Clozapine	Clozaril	300-900 mg
Molindone	Moban	20-225 mg
Perphenazine	Trilafon	8-60 mg
Loxapine	Loxitane	50-250 mg
Trifluoperazine	Stelazine	10-40 mg
Fluphenazine	Prolixin	3-45 mg
Thiothixene	Navane	10-60 mg
Haloperidol	Haldol	2-40 mg

Adapted and used with permission from *Handbook of Clinical Psychopharmacology for Therapists* by John D. Preston, John O'Neil, and Mary Talaga. Oakland, CA: New Harbinger Publications, 1994.

By the end of the second day at home, Melissa was feeling strange. She could not sit still and paced for an hour at a time. When she slept, she slept fitfully, and had frightening dreams. She repeatedly thought she saw something dash across the floor, out of the corner of her eye. When she turned to look, she could see nothing. She mentioned none of this to her husband, Tony, who only noticed that Melissa seemed exhausted.

By the morning of her fourth day at home, Melissa was hallucinating. She wakened her husband at 6:20, screaming and wailing that the baby was Jesus Christ, come to take her sins away. She was waving the baby through the air, chanting about him being able to fly. Her husband grabbed the baby and called 911. Emergency personnel came and transported Melissa, Tony, and the baby to the local hospital. Melissa was admitted to the psychiatric unit, and her husband learned that she was suffering from postpartum psychosis. She was administered *Thorazine*, with *Cogentin* to control the side effects. As she had been breastfeeding, the baby had to be weaned suddenly. But the doctor reassured Tony that everything would be fine. It was lucky that Tony had been home at the time, and was able to get Melissa to the hospital before she harmed herself or the baby.

Melissa was stable on the medication after about 72 hours, and was released from the hospital two days after that. She remained on the medication for about nine months, and then slowly tapered off. She also received counseling. Melissa was sad about having had to wean the baby so suddenly; she'd always planned to breastfeed her baby longer. She also felt some guilt and shame about "having gone off the deep end" after her baby was born. But in counseling she learned to accept that the psychotic episode had been purely biochemical, and couldn't in any way be seen to be her fault. She went on to become a wonderful mother and to have a great relationship with her baby.

Anti-mania Medications

When a postpartum woman is suffering from mania, she may have

- Decreased need for sleep
- Rapid and pressured speech
- Racing thoughts
- Distractibility
- Irritability
- Increased activity
- Poor judgment

She may seem to be running at a million miles an hour. It may be difficult to interrupt her speech. She may feel she can accomplish anything, but will actually finish very little. Lithium is the primary medication used to treat manic symptoms, although MAO inhibitors (see section on antidepressants) and *Tegretol* (carbamazepine, an antiseizure drug) are sometimes used as well. Daily dosages of lithium generally range from 1200 to 3000 mg, after starting with doses of 600 to 900 mg/day. Lithium can control the symptoms, and prevent recurrence or relapse. Often a physician will begin treatment with both lithium and an antipsychotic medication, in order to control the symptoms more quickly. The antipsychotic drug is then phased out when the lithium kicks in.

When a patient is taking lithium, the level of the drug in the bloodstream must be closely monitored. This is because the level required for the drug to work is very close to the level at which toxicity, or poisoning, can occur. Lithium has a number of major side effects, many of which can be avoided by taking divided doses, or will subside as time passes. The signs of lithium toxicity, and the side effects, should be thoroughly explained to you by your prescribing physician. Lithium is not addictive, and is perfectly safe if closely monitored.

Lithium is sometimes administered in low doses as an addition to antidepressant medications. The blood level may again need to be watched closely. Careful monitoring can make the difference between antidepressants giving relief and not working at all.

Rosemary was a 27-year-old nurse. When she gave birth to her first baby, her husband was overseas with his military unit. Rosemary and the baby were living with her in-laws. Everything went well for the first ten days. Then June, Rosemary's mother-in-law, noticed that Rosemary didn't seem to be sleeping at all. When June awakened at 3 a.m. to take her turn at feeding the baby, she found Rosemary jogging on the minitrampoline in the den. June asked her if she was okay, to which Rosemary snapped irritably that she "just needed her exercise."

The next day, June shared her concerns with Joe, her husband. He thought this was probably just Rosemary's attempts to regain her figure. By that afternoon, though, Rosemary was buzzing around the house, first mopping the floor, then scrubbing the tub with bleach, all the time talking nonstop about "protecting the baby from germs." This went on for two more days before June became more concerned and called Rosemary's doctor. The nurse who took the call had an aunt with manic-depressive illness, and recognized Rosemary's symptoms. She recommended that June take Rosemary right away to see a psychiatrist.

June called a friend who had a sister who was a psychiatrist, and promptly made an appointment for the next day. Rosemary balked at the idea, reassuring her mother-in-law that she just felt "antsy" from being cooped up in the house with the baby. Joe had to help June load Rosemary into the car for the appointment. In the doctor's office, Rosemary paced and paced, unable to sit still. The psychiatrist diagnosed a postpartum manic reaction, and prescribed lithium. She recommended hospitalization, but Rosemary rejected the idea completely. On the doctor's advice, Joe and June took turns sitting up with Rosemary, closely watching her over several days, until the lithium began to calm her.

As her symptoms subsided Rosemary could see that her behavior had been odd. She felt better on the medication, and felt able to cooperate with the rest of her treatment knowing that it would allow her to do a good job caring for her baby. She had several sessions of counseling with the psychiatrist, helping her to accept that her behavior had been biochemically related and not due to her failure as a person or a parent. After about a year, she was able to taper off the medication without problems.

Sleep Medications

Sleep problems are a common symptom in many postpartum reactions. Many women find that the self-care strategies for solving these sleep problems just do not provide enough relief. A new mother's anxiety about insomnia may build as she wonders how she will get through the next day—how she'll be able to care for the baby or function at her job—if she doesn't get some sleep. As this anxiety about sleep builds, so does her insomnia: it can become harder and harder to fall asleep. When this vicious cycle seems to take on a life of its own, medication may be needed.

Some physicians will recommend *Benadryl,* an over-the-counter allergy medication, as the first sleep aid to try. The sleepiness caused by this drug can sometimes avoid the need for a prescription medication. Be sure to check with your physician before trying *Benadryl* as a sleep aid. According to Kathleen Huggins, author of *The Nursing Mother's Companion, Benadryl* does pass through the breastmilk, and at dosages above 25mg/day may cause drowsiness in your baby.

Anti-anxiety medication can often interrupt the anxiety cycle that prevents sleep. Antidepressant medication often works to induce sleep as well. A certain class of anti-anxiety medications—the benzodiazepine sedative hypnotics—can be an effective, safe way to interrupt the insomnia cycle. These drugs are targeted directly at the sleep problem, rather than at the other anxiety or depression symptoms. These drugs and their usual dosages are listed in the chart below.

Sleep Medications

Generic Name	Brand Name	Usual Daily Dosage
Flurazepam	*Dalmane*	15-30 mg
Temazepam	*Restoril*	15-30 mg
Triazolam	*Halcion*	.25-.5 mg
Quazepam	*Doral*	7.5-15 mg
Estazolam	*ProSom*	1-2 mg
Zolpidem	*Ambien*	10-20 mg

Adapted and used with permission from *Clinical Psychopharmacology Made Ridiculously Simple* by John Preston and James Johnson. Miami: MedMaster, Inc., 1993.

Carrie was a 33-year-old flight attendant. She did well in the first six weeks postpartum, while she was off work. When she returned to flying, however, she had significant trouble falling asleep. Her problems began when she was away from the baby on an overnight layover in a distant city. She could not fall asleep, worrying about the baby at home, and wondering how her husband was faring alone. On her first overnight, she only got three hours of sleep before she had to get up to fly back home. Then the same thing happened at home. She could not get back to sleep, no matter what she tried, after waking to feed the baby her 2 a.m. bottle. Carrie worried that she would not be able to function on the next day's flight. Sure enough, the next day she was very groggy, and spilled a meal in a first-class passenger's lap! She was mortified, and slept even less the next two nights, one of them away and one at home.

Carrie had ten days of the insomnia before she called her company doctor. After a brief consultation, the doctor prescribed *Restoril*, to be taken at bedtime. The medication made her very drowsy, and she went right to sleep. After about four nights of catching up, Carrie tried going to sleep without the drug. It was a little more difficult than with the medicine, but Carrie did manage to fall asleep on her own. She was a bit concerned about becoming too dependent on the drug. When she discussed this with the doctor, he reassured her that, if she only took it when she really needed it, she would not become dependent. Carrie continued to take the drug two or three times a week for about six weeks, and then found that she had tapered off to not needing it at all.

Hormone Intervention

There is considerable controversy surrounding the use of hormones, particularly progesterone and estrogen, to treat postpartum emotional reactions. Dr. Katharina Dalton, a British physician and author of *Depression After Childbirth*, has been a long-time advocate of using natural (not synthetic) progesterone to treat and/or prevent postpartum depression. Dr. Dalton writes that the administration of considerable doses of progesterone in the postpartum period cushions the normal abrupt decline in progesterone after the birth of a baby. With this gentler drop in the hormone level, she feels that many symptoms can be prevented, as the woman's hormone level returns to prepregnancy levels more gradually. In addition, progesterone inhibits monoamine oxidase activity (MAO), acting like the MAO inhibitors that are used as antidepressants. There are many physicians and their patients who feel that progesterone treatment is highly effective. Physicians are more apt to offer progesterone therapy because they feel it is natural, does not interfere with breastfeeding, and does little harm. Often though, the dosage physicians prescribe is too low, and so may not be helpful.

Dr. Dalton's claims about the value of progesterone therapy have not been supported by research in the United States. When large-scale research studies compared those women who received progesterone with those women who received a placebo (a pill without any active therapeutic ingredients), the two groups did not seem to differ in their reaction. Because the groups of women taking progesterone didn't feel better sooner, many physicians in this country reject the idea of prescribing it for postpartum depression. Some physicians even feel it can be harmful, in that a woman may suffer needlessly before using a more effective medication.

How can you make sense of this controversy and decide what to do for yourself? In our practice as psychologists, we have seen numerous women benefit from progesterone therapy. We feel that it should be considered on a case-by-case basis. You need to evaluate the controversy with the aid of your health-care practitioners, and together decide what is best for you. The fact that progesterone can be used without jeopardizing breastfeeding is important, and so deserves consideration.

In our clinical work, it appears that there may be certain subtypes of postpartum women for whom progesterone therapy is effective. We've found that women with anxiety-related postpartum reactions, rather than depression, seem to respond well to progesterone. We have seen progesterone therapy work well with women with mania, panic, and obsessive-compulsive reactions. It does not seem to work as well with women whose main symptoms are crying, sleeping too much, inability to get dressed, and just down-in-the-dumps depression. It's possible that large-scale research studies have not been dividing women into groups according to subtypes of emotional reactions. If the women with depression, mania, obsessive thoughts, and panic are all lumped together in one big group for research purposes, that might explain the lack of positive effect for progesterone therapy. More detailed and refined research protocols are needed before more definitive answers are available about the value of progesterone therapy.

In women in the anxiety subcategory mentioned above, therapy must be done correctly. The treatment must be started quickly. The more days pass after the birth of the baby, the less likely it is that the progesterone will help. Ideally, progesterone can be administered (as an injection, suppository, or sublingual tablet) on the birthing bed, and may be best suited for prevention at this point when a woman has a history of postpartum reactions. The dose must be sufficiently large to get a response. Your physician can get dosage information from any of the nationally accessible women's pharmacies which compound natural progesterone. You can find information in the Resources Section for locating these pharmacies.

Karen had her first child when she was 29. She experienced a mild postpartum reaction: she was anxious, and worried a great deal about whether she had "done the right thing" by having a baby. By making some lifestyle changes, and switching her focus from work to home, she began to feel that motherhood "fit" her after all.

Even though she was still breastfeeding the baby, at four months postpartum Karen began to have menstrual spotting or breakthrough bleeding, preceding her period each month. The bleeding increased to where she bled for about 10 days out of every 28-day cycle. Karen felt tired, and figured she was anemic from the blood loss, but didn't pursue any testing or treatment.

When their first child was three, Karen and George decided to have another baby. After six months of trying Karen went to her doctor. The blood samples and endometrial biopsy showed that she had "luteal phase deficiency." Inadequate progesterone in her system kept the lining of her uterus from building up sufficiently each month for a fertilized egg to implant there. Karen's doctor prescribed progesterone suppositories and *Clomid*, a fertility drug. Karen became pregnant the very next month (fortunately with a single baby). Karen and George were thrilled! With the birth of the new baby, Karen was again troubled by anxiety and irritability. Neither she not her doctor made the connection to the progesterone problem and Karen "toughed it out." Then the spotting began again, and when her menstrual cycle resumed, she found herself faced with rampant premenstrual syndrome (PMS). For two weeks every month, she would be irritable, have sleep difficulties, yell at everyone, and feel a "sinking" feeling about her life in general. Her nearly constant bleeding became increasingly troublesome as well. Karen went through several doctors, trying to find an answer: from her obstetrician to an endocrinologist to a psychiatrist. The endocrinologist prescribed progesterone suppositories, to use the last 14 days of her cycle.

The first month was delightful; Karen felt remarkably less cranky and irritable. And she was even more amazed to find that the progesterone had shortened her period to four days of bleeding! After four months on the suppositories, Karen found that she was free not just from the debilitating emotions, but from her physical symptoms of excessive bleeding as well.

Besides progesterone, medical researchers around the United States are beginning to try estrogen as a treatment for postpartum emotional reactions. Deborah Sichel, M.D., and Lee Cohen, M.D., of Massachusetts General Hospital Perinatal Psychiatry Clinical Research Program in Boston, have had several successes using estrogen with postpartum psychosis. Similarly, M.E. Ted Quigley, M.D., who is Clinical Associate Professor of Endocrinology at the University of California at San Diego, has used testosterone, progesterone, and estrogen to treat postpartum depression, with positive results. Addresses and phone numbers for these researchers can be found in the Resources Section.

Breastfeeding and Medications

Until recently, there appeared to be no debate about whether a breastfeeding woman could take psychotropic medications. The answer was a clear and resounding "no." It was assumed that the drug would enter the breastmilk, and the baby would then be receiving it as well. Even now, most physicians will give this negative answer if you ask them about taking antidepressants while continuing to nurse your baby.

Currently, however, research by several groups across the country is suggesting that there are some circumstances and some medications that *are* compatible with breastfeeding. Deborah Sichel, M.D., and Lee Cohen, M.D., of the Perinatal Psychiatry Clinical Research Program at Massachusetts General Hospital, and Katherine Wisner, M.D., M.S., of Mood Disorders Program, Case Western Reserve University, Cleveland, have been researching this topic with fairly promising results. These physicians have studied the levels of specific drugs, both in the breastmilk and in the blood of breastfeeding infants.

Based on this research, antidepressant medications that appear to be acceptable (if a mother must take medication and wishes to continue breastfeeding) are nortriptyline, imiprimine, and desiprimine. These researchers have found mixed results when studying fluoxetine. With clomiprimine, higher levels of the drug have been found in the breastmilk than with the drugs mentioned above. Carbamazepine (*Tegretol*) does not seem to show up in the breastmilk either, and so may be an acceptable medication for the postpartum woman with manic symptoms.

Neuroleptics—usually called antipsychotic medications—may be used with breastfeeding mothers who suffer from mania or psychosis. According to the Marcé Society, an international organization devoted to the study of prenatal and postpartum mental health, these medications do enter the milk in small quantities, but there is no evidence in recent research that they affect the infant adversely. The Marcé Society is launching a widespread study of the use of these drugs with postpartum psychosis, and will likely have further information about these drugs and breastfeeding in the future.

There is little information at this time about anti-anxiety medication and breastfeeding. Research has indicated that lithium, diazepam (*Valium*), and doxepin (an antidepressant) are not compatible with breastfeeding, as too much of these medications passes into the baby's blood via the mother's breastmilk.

Drs. Cohen, Sichel, and Wisner all require that mothers who wish to take antidepressant medications and breastfeed have regular lab tests to examine the levels of the drug in their breastmilk, and have the baby's blood tested as well. If you wish to attempt taking such medications and continuing to breastfeed, you need to ask your doctor and the baby's pediatrician to arrange for these tests. You'll also want to discuss the issue with your child's pediatrician. These precautions are extremely important, for, as the researchers point out, the levels of the medication detected in the breastmilk are extremely variable, depending on different factors, including time of day. To be safe, both your milk and the baby's blood should be monitored carefully. Dr. Cohen recommends testing both the breastmilk and the baby's blood when the baby is seven to ten days old, and at regular intervals after that. Dr. Wisner recommends extreme caution with newborns, and reports that she is much more likely to prescribe antidepressants for the mother of a two- to three-month-old baby.

As always, deciding to take medication while breastfeeding should be discussed with your own physician as well as your child's pediatrician. You need to carefully weigh any risks to the baby against the benefits to your recovery. This is not a decision to be taken lightly, as there is no long-term data available: it is only since 1989 that mothers have attempted to breastfeed while on antidepressants. Any long-term effects may not yet be evident, even with trace amounts of drug in the breastmilk. We present this information here to help you and your physician make this decision on an individual basis. For the latest results, you may want your physician to contact the doctors listed above. Their addresses, again, are in the Resources Section.

8

Weathering the Storm:
Three Stories of Recovery

A Brief Note of Encouragement,
Because This Chapter Can't
Be Summarized Very Well

If you or someone close to you is experiencing a postpartum reaction, you may be wondering, "How long can this go on?" In
response to your difficulties, you may be feeling helpless or hopeless or both. You may be sad or angry that having a child did
not match your expectations; you may question, "Why me?" Perhaps you feel let down by God or fate; perhaps you grieve your
lost dreams. The proverbial light at the end of the tunnel may
look pretty dim just now. Sometimes there may seem to be no
light at all. Facing each day may be a challenge that you feel less
and less able to meet. And through all of this, you may be asking
yourself, "Will my life ever be okay again? When will my pain
and suffering end? How long will it take me to get better?"

You will get better, but there is no one easy answer we can give about the length of time it will take you to recover. Every postpartum reaction, and every woman, is different. Change occurs step by step. At first, change may hardly seem noticeable at all. But it does come; it's just hard to see because it's incremental. Do you remember how dramatically your friends' babies seemed to change from week to week, or month to month, before you had a baby of your own? Isn't it hard to see your own baby growing and changing when the changes come so gradually, day by day? Because you're with *yourself* every day, it's difficult to register the changes and progress you're making. But if you were an outsider looking in—if you didn't see yourself for a week or a month at a time—the changes would be dramatic and unmistakable. You *are* making progress, but you may just have to take it on faith for a while.

Follow through with the suggestions and guidelines in this book. Pursue one small goal at a time. Then go on to another. If you're working with one or more helping professionals, listen to them. Follow their advice if it seems sensible to you. Be persistent in your belief that you can and will feel well again. Recovery is a process; it takes time. Repeat this to yourself whenever you run out of steam and feel that you can't go one step further. Trust that you can get better; that you can heal.

This chapter tells the story of three women who successfully recovered from their postpartum reactions. Although their experiences may be different from yours, there will also be similarities. Each of these new moms questioned whether she would ever get through her postpartum agony. Like you, each of them struggled with many painful emotions. As you read their stories, think about the coping strategies they used to survive their experience. You may want to review your current recovery plan, and see whether you want to make any changes based on what you learn from these women. But, whatever you decide, don't measure your recovery by their experiences. For every new mom, the postpartum recovery process is unique. Go at your own pace, and follow your own signposts.

Every woman who journeys through a postpartum reaction is a survivor. Pat yourself on the back for having come this far. And then keep moving forward. Health and peace of mind await you at the end of the tunnel.

Exercise
Two Minutes for Yourself

Because there is so much uncertainty in life, and especially in having a baby, you may find yourself worrying about many things. From your child's health and development, to fears about kidnappers or earthquakes or fires, to whether your child will want to ride a motorcycle as a teenager, worries can consume you.

Instead of spending your energy on circumstances and situations that are largely beyond your control, reel in your imagination and focus on what you can do to make your child's life as safe, fulfilled, and happy as possible. Answer every worry with a calming thought. This exercise will show you how.

Take a sheet of paper, or a page in a notebook, and divide it into two columns. Label one column *Worried Thoughts*, and the other *Calming Thoughts*. Carry this, and a pencil or pen, with you wherever you go. Whenever a worried thought pops into your head, write it down. If a calming thought occurs to you right away, write this down, too. For instance, if your thought was, "I'll never get organized. Look at this messy house!", your calming response might be, "Houses with infants in them are almost always disorganized. Relax! You can make a list and start to get things done one at a time."

If you can't think of a calming thought to answer one of your worries, try to imagine that you're not you, but a dear and kind and supportive friend of yours. It doesn't matter if that person is real or just a friend you'd like to have. Now look at your unanswered worry again. What would your friend say to soothe you? Close your eyes and listen. Then write down her words in the calming thoughts column.

Worries are a part of motherhood, but they don't have to dominate your view. Spend some time every day reading just the *Calming Thoughts* column of your list. Dwell on those calming thoughts. Rehearse them in your head. Say them out loud. Sing them to your baby. Practice thinking them, breathing slowly and deeply, until they come as second nature to you.

8

Weathering the Storm:
Three Stories of Recovery

Karen's Story

After three years of marriage, 30-year-old Karen and her 26-year-old husband Jim decided to "take the plunge" into parenthood. She was working as a clerk in a small accounting firm; Jim worked second shift in the elevator repair department of a large hospital complex. Karen and Jim had worked hard in the first part of their marriage to divide up the housework duties equally, and discussed how they would share parenting duties equally as well. They seemed to be launched into the parenting world quite quickly: after only two months of trying to get pregnant, they succeeded. The pregnancy went smoothly, with Karen feeling well and Jim quite proud of his "budding" wife. They talked about everything, and felt as prepared as they could be. The nursery was set up, the plan for Karen to take an extended leave of absence laid out. Jim would work on call at his job for extra family income while Karen was off work. They were both committed to Karen breastfeeding their baby. Jim's schedule allowed him to attend Karen's prenatal doctor visits with her. It was a surprise to them both how little worry or anxiety they felt about this grand upcoming event.

Thirteen days before her due date, Karen was surprised to wake up soaked at 3 a.m. She shook Jim with great excitement. "My water broke, this must be it!" she told him. Jim called the doctor while Karen took a shower. The doctor told them to come on in to the hospital, which they did like two children on their way to the candy store. They arrived at the labor and delivery room almost giddy with excitement, with Karen's contractions coming about four minutes apart. It was the night before the Fourth of July. They soon found that the maternity ward was understaffed because of the holiday, and the nurses who had pulled this unattractive holiday duty were none too happy to be there. A series of unpleasant events ensued, with Karen getting more irritated and exhausted as the night progressed. She was denied an enema on the grounds that the nurse had felt her bowel area and said there was "nothing there." Karen and Jim were mortified about the result of that later, during the baby's birth when the nurses grumbled about Karen having "made a mess of the delivery table."

But finally, after a heroic labor with no medication, their baby boy was born at 11:50 a.m. Karen and Jim were jubilant. They named him Ryan James. They got to hold him for about 45 minutes in the recovery room, and then he was taken to the nursery while Karen was moved to her room. She had requested rooming-in, and was told she would have to wait for about three hours. It was now early afternoon, so Karen decided to try and catch a nap before the baby was brought to her, while Jim went off to call friends and family. She napped fitfully, wondering when they'd bring her baby to her. By 5 p.m. she called the nursery and asked that Ryan be brought to her room. She was told that he was "not yet ready." Karen continued to call every half hour, requesting her baby for breastfeeding, and was put off each time, being told that the nurses were "too busy." Karen and Jim were getting madder and madder! How could they get going on breastfeeding if the nurses wouldn't bring the baby? At 7:30 that evening, Jim couldn't take any more, and went down to the nursery and brought back the baby himself. The night in the hospital went more smoothly after that, with Jim and Karen taking turns holding Ryan for the entire night. He began to nurse fairly well, and they sighed a big sigh of relief, feeling back on track with their well-made plans.

Karen's nursing care continued to suffer because of the holiday weekend, however. She asked repeatedly for a pitcher of water to quench her thirst, but she only got one glass at a time, with hours in between. She did not receive the bottle for cleansing her perineum that her doctor mentioned, either. Karen and Jim had asked, in advance, to be present when Ryan was circumcised. Somehow this was neglected as well. They had planned to attend the baby-care classes offered by the hospital, which would instruct them on changing and bathing the baby and caring for his umbilical cord. But because of the holiday, there was no class. Finally, their pediatrician told them that they would receive a booklet on baby care when they checked out. When Karen got home from the hospital, she couldn't find this booklet in her bag or among any of her possessions.

Jim could not remember having received it at all, so they called the hospital and spoke to the head nurse. Checking Karen's chart, the nurse told her that Karen had signed the checkout checklist saying that she had been given the booklet. When Karen protested, the nurse told her she must have been too heavily medicated to remember. But Karen hadn't had any medication, and Jim couldn't remember having received the booklet either.

It was a relief to be home and away from such rudeness and incompetence. Jim took three days off from work so that he could be at home with Karen and Ryan. The first couple of days went fairly smoothly, although Karen had little experience with babies, and felt at a loss about what to do when Ryan cried. It was all so foreign to her! She had never even babysat a newborn. "Why couldn't we have gone to the baby classes?" she obsessed. Maybe then she would have felt like a competent parent. Fortunately, Jim had three young nieces who lived in town. He had often taken care of them, even as infants, giving his sister much-needed relief. He felt quite confident as a parent. As Karen became more and more flustered, Jim decided it would be best to take an "instructor" role with her. He held a "miniclass" on baby-care basics for Karen, showing her how to burp, change, and even bathe Ryan. After that, the routine of nurse, nap, change the baby, nurse, nap, change the baby blended the days and nights together—but the fog was a pleasant one. On her third day at home, Karen was suddenly running a fever of 103.3. Jim called the doctor, who arranged to see her that afternoon.

Karen had developed an infection in her episiotomy. The good news was that it was treatable by antibiotics. The bad news was that she couldn't continue to breastfeed while taking the prescribed drugs. Tender, sore, and bitterly disappointed, she returned home in tears. As Karen lay in bed sobbing, Jim, juggling Ryan on his shoulder, called their childbirth educator. After Jim explained the situation, she gave him the name of a lactation consultant who could help Karen. The consultant came over that same evening with a rented breast pump, and talked with Karen and Jim about what they could do to sustain Karen's milk supply until her week on antibiotics was over.

Not breastfeeding made Karen feel totally disconnected from baby Ryan. Nursing was how she had defined being the mother of an infant! She cried and talked with Jim, who also felt disappointed. It was only a week, he tried to console her. There were certainly other ways to parent—after all, he wasn't breastfeeding, and he was still a parent. Nevertheless, Karen decided she must get up at every feeding to feed Ryan his formula. She could not let Jim do even one feeding, even though she had to pump her breasts as well. Discouraged but resigned, Jim went back to work. He actually felt relieved to be back to a regular routine, as he was pretty tired of getting up at night anyway. He had never functioned well on less than eight hours of sleep.

So, for three days, Karen did it all. She was getting more and more exhausted. "But how can I do anything else?" she thought. "This is my baby, who I looked forward to for so long." Karen had always been prone to worry. Now she found herself thinking that she was a failure as a mom. This parent stuff was not all it was cracked up to be. Sure, Ryan was sweet—she loved the moments when he was curled up on her chest, sleeping peacefully. But to be up every three hours, all night long; or the time he screamed for 45 minutes without stopping—these experiences left her feeling as if all of this had been a *big* mistake. By the third night of solo parenting Karen began to feel funny while Jim was at work. Her chest hurt, she had trouble breathing, and she felt clammy and sweaty. She didn't realize she was having a panic attack. When Jim came home, she told him about her difficulties. He thought she was probably just exhausted. It was more than that, she insisted. She felt nauseous much of the time. She felt incredibly scatterbrained, after always being so organized and precise. They talked until 3 a.m., and he convinced her to let his mother, who lived nearby, take Ryan for several days so that Karen could get caught up on her sleep. She would still have to pump her breasts, but it would be much easier to do so without trying to keep Ryan happy at the same time. Reluctantly, Karen let Jim take Ryan to his grandparents the next morning. She felt a bit ready for a break.

With Ryan gone, Karen slept the entire next day. She awoke after ten hours, her breasts aching and engorged from not using the pump. She expressed her breastmilk, had some dinner, and went back to bed. She awoke in a sweat after three hours, having dreamt that Ryan was floating away from her on a swirling river. Every time she closed her eyes, this picture returned. By midnight, when Jim returned from work, Karen was anxious and agitated. She was feeling panicky again, and had been unable to sleep. Jim turned on some of their favorite music, sat Karen down on the couch with him, and rubbed her shoulders for 30 minutes. They avoided talking about Karen's problems; Jim told her "just don't think about it!" every time she tried to voice her concerns. She was finally able to sleep, for another nine hours straight. By the time two nights had gone by, Karen was ready for Ryan to come home again. She felt more rested and a bit more confident about giving this mothering business another try.

Karen and Jim brought Ryan home the next day. Karen was finished with the antibiotics now, and was delighted to resume nursing her baby. But the first day of this turned out to be a nightmare. Jim was at work, so Karen was at home again on her own with the baby. She nursed Ryan for an hour, after which he finally drifted off to sleep, only to jerk awake, rooting for her breast, 20 minutes later. This went on for most of the day. Karen felt like one big nipple. During one nursing session, the baby stayed latched on for nearly three hours! She couldn't get him to sleep for more than 30 minutes. Every time she tried to pull him gently away from her breast, he would awaken screaming and rooting again. Nothing calmed him but having her nipple in his mouth.

When Jim came home, he gave Ryan a big bottle of formula, and Ryan slept for five hours straight. Karen was relieved at first, but finally awakened in a panic again, worrying when Ryan would wake up and resume his fussing and screaming. The next day was a repeat, with Ryan fussing and sleeping fitfully and Karen basically nursing him all day long. The following morning Karen was in tears as she and Jim talked about what to do. She was feeling like a failure as a mother again. Jim suggested there was a pattern, with Ryan doing well once he had a bottle of formula. Perhaps Ryan was simply hungry. He suggested they call the lactation consultant Carol again, which Karen did. Carol agreed that Ryan was probably not getting enough breastmilk, and was quite likely hungry, given their description of the problem. They made an appointment for Carol to come observe Ryan breastfeeding the next day, to rule out any problems with latching on or sucking.

Watching Ryan at the breast, Carol felt that his technique was fine, and Karen appeared quite confident in her handling of him. Carol explained that nursing is a supply-and-demand system. Ryan probably wasn't getting enough to eat because Karen's milk supply had been compromised when Ryan stayed with Jim's mother. With her need to catch up on her sleep, Karen hadn't pumped her breasts frequently enough to signal her breasts to maintain their production at full swing. Ryan's demanding appetite was his way of trying to get Karen to step up production to meet his needs.

Carol was able to provide Karen with a device called a nursing supplementer, which would augment Ryan's intake of milk while stimulating Karen's breasts to produce more milk. The device was a plastic bottle with thin latex tubes coming out of it. Karen was to fill the bottle with formula, wear it on a string around her neck, and tape the tubes to her nipples. When Ryan nursed, he got some of the formula as well as whatever breastmilk Karen was producing. As she taught Karen how to use the device, and showed her how to tape the ends of the tubes in place, Carol complimented Karen on how relaxed she seemed as a mother.

That did it! The floodgates opened, and Karen's tears rushed out. She did not feel confident, she wailed. Those first two weeks had been a nightmare. The breastfeeding was all a mess, she couldn't sleep, she felt like a failure wearing this horrible gadget and having to give her baby formula because she couldn't even produce enough milk for him on her own. She lamented the fiasco parenting had felt like for her, telling about her nausea, her worries, her panic. Carol gave Karen a hug as she continued to sob. Carol made Karen sit down on the couch, brought her a glass of juice, and rocked the baby to sleep while Karen settled down. Carol gently told Karen that she thought she might be suffering from some postpartum depression, brought on by the physical and emotional stresses of the birth and all the new challenges of parenting. She recommended that Karen talk with her physician, as well as with a psychologist specializing in postpartum adjustment issues. Carol would provide support and encouragement on rebuilding Karen's milk production so that she might at least feel like a success with the nursing.

When Jim came home that evening, Karen filled him in on her meeting with Carol. He listened, and readily agreed to Carol's idea about calling Karen's doctor first. After all, they knew and trusted him. Maybe they could avoid going to a psychologist if the OB could give them some ideas on what would help. So Karen called her doctor the next morning. After meeting with her, he agreed with the lactation consultant that Karen seemed to be suffering from postpartum depression. His recommendation was that Karen get on an antidepressant as well as an anti-anxiety medication. Karen's heart sank when the doctor said that she couldn't continue to breastfeed on the medication. She hung up the phone and sank onto the couch next to Jim, dissolving into tears again. How could she give up the breastfeeding, after all this struggle? She was just getting going on that again! Jim put his arm around her and held her, feeling helpless. This was all feeling like too much to him.

Then Karen suddenly perked up. "I could still call the psychologist!" she said. Carol had told her that the psychologist did not prescribe medication. Maybe there *was* another option. She called the psychologist right away, and got the answering service. When the operator asked if it was an emergency, Karen burst into tears again. Through her sobs she gave her name and number, and said that she had hoped the doctor could call back right away. Ten minutes later, the phone rang. Karen told the psychologist her story, and the psychologist listened intently, interrupting only once in a while to ask questions. She told Karen that it sounded as if she did, indeed, have a postpartum emotional reaction; but she reassured her that many women dealt with such difficulties without medication. It made sense, she thought, to try other interventions first. Karen made an appointment for the next day, feeling much relieved. "I couldn't believe someone sounded so understanding." The psychologist had sounded so supportive about breastfeeding, and seemed to know exactly where Karen was coming from.

Leaving the baby with Jim the next day, Karen went to see the psychologist. She felt a bit nervous, but was also more optimistic than she'd been since Ryan's birth. In the first session, she was able to relax a great deal as she told her story. The doctor reassured her that many women have similar feelings after the birth of a baby. As Karen talked, she became aware of how much she felt that Jim had been pulling away from her in this trouble. She suddenly realized that he seemed to want to put the baby off on his parents as the answer to Karen's every concern. Karen found that she was suddenly very angry at Jim, and felt that he was not holding up his end of the parenting job. The psychologist helped Karen see that Jim's actions and attitudes were also a common reaction to a new baby, and pointed out that maybe Jim felt as insecure as she did. He simply showed it in a different way.

By the end of the session, Karen had a list of things she could do in the next week to feel better. She was going to take a rest every day, and do one fun thing each day as well. She was going to take a short walk every evening. The doctor had recommended that she use the front pack to carry Ryan, both on walks and to do such household tasks as vacuuming, because babies who are carried more frequently actually cry less. And because Karen felt that she was spinning her wheels, getting little accomplished each day, she was to keep a running tally of every baby-care task she got done. This way, she would see that she actually was getting much done, even though her accomplishments might not be as visible as the backlog of household chores. Finally, Karen was going to bring Jim with her the next week, to involve him in her process of feeling better, and give them a chance to discuss her newly discovered anger about how *he* was adjusting to parenting.

That first week, Karen began to feel like there was indeed "light at the end of the tunnel." She tried the things that had been suggested in that first session. Getting rest and a bit of exercise certainly helped, and Ryan did seem to cry less when he was carried more. She still had to use the nursing supplementer, and felt like a failure each time she clipped the bottle onto the string around her neck. But she tried to tune in to how she was succeeding. She did feel better taking time to read the comics each day; that was fun, and goodness knows she had had little fun since Ryan was born. Karen was so mad, now that she had recognized Jim's distancing. He was signing up for every extra shift and "on-call" slot that he could. She realized they had discussed this before the baby was born, and she knew it was his way of trying to "provide" and be a good father. But, practically speaking, it meant that Karen and Ryan were home alone from noon to nearly midnight six days of the week. That didn't feel like the "equal" parenting that Karen and Jim had planned during pregnancy.

Karen was trying to keep a lid on her anger, and to wait for the next appointment before talking about this issue with Jim. But then, two days before the appointment, when Jim was supposed to be taking care of Ryan, Karen returned from her walk to find the baby fussing in the swing while Jim lounged in the recliner, watching a baseball game on TV. Karen just blew up. Jim jumped up as soon as he saw her, insisting that Ryan had only begun to fuss. But Karen could tell from Ryan's red face that he'd been crying longer than "just a minute." She called Jim a "lousy father" and said she couldn't even trust him with the baby. If he'd been a sitter, she would have fired him on the spot. A yelling match followed, with Jim and Karen both saying many hurtful things about each other's value as a parent and a person. Jim finally slammed out the door to go to work, and Karen collapsed on the couch in tears once again. They did not speak during the entire two days until the next appointment.

Jim and Karen walked into the psychologist's office an angry, sulky couple. When the doctor asked Jim why he was there, he retorted that he wasn't sure—he'd like to be anywhere else. The only way the psychologist could get them to talk to each other was about what baby Ryan needed: it was obvious that they were both intently focused on their baby. The doctor began by telling Jim about the prevalence of postpartum depression and panic, and how it isn't the woman's or the couple's fault, but rather arises from a combination of stressors, physical and biological. When Jim realized he was not going to be blamed, he began to relax and talk about how hard this whole process had been on him. He had felt well-prepared, because of his experience with infants. But he was scared by his resentment of the baby, and his wishes that Ryan had never appeared in their lives. When the psychologist identified these concerns as quite normal, Jim felt less guilty.

As Karen listened to her husband talk, she became aware of how painful all of this was for him, too. It had been hard to remember this when she was the one at home with the baby, all alone, day after day. This phrase—"all alone, day after day"—had come up repeatedly in their conversations, and the doctor pointed this out. Karen began to cry again. "It's true—I *feel* so alone!" It became clear that Karen needed more contact with other mothers, as well as more breaks from her "on-duty" time. For the next week, the couple negotiated a plan: Jim would give Karen 30 minutes of time each morning before he went to work, to do something on her own while he was completely "in charge" of Ryan. Karen was going to continue to try to exercise, rest, and have some fun. And she was going to try to make contact with some other mothers who had infants, to relieve her feeling of being alone. She had been planning to attend a breastfeeding support group, and promised herself to make that a priority.

Karen and Ryan attended the support group next week, and Karen greatly enjoyed the contact with other mothers. One of the mothers who had an older child had held Ryan for the whole meeting, simply wanting to hold an infant. Karen found that to be the most helpful relief she had felt in weeks. But things did not go so smoothly between Karen and Jim. He didn't take the initiative for giving her the much-needed break time each day, but rather did it only if she insisted, and then complained that he had "too much to do." When Karen and Jim came in for their next therapy appointment, it became clear that housework had been a long-standing struggle between them. This was now amplified by the added burden of infant care. Jim was perfectly content to have Karen plop Ryan in his lap as he watched TV each morning, but Karen wanted him to interact more with Ryan. The same was true for household chores: Jim was very willing to do them, but at his own pace and using his own standards and methods. They became aware that they had very different ideas about how to do these chores and take care of the baby.

The psychologist helped them see that they could find some middle ground. Karen made some specific requests of Jim, that he ask every day, "How can I help you today?" and that he smile and try not to sigh when she handed him the baby. He admitted that his previous reactions probably would have bothered him if he had been Karen; he hadn't realized how sour he'd been. The couple also talked about how tired they both were, getting up so frequently with the baby, who seemed to take more than an hour to go back to sleep after his nighttime feedings. The doctor recommended that they not stay up with Ryan at those times, but that they lay him back in his crib still awake, as long as he did not cry for more than a few minutes. She stressed that babies need to learn to fall asleep on their own, and parents can help them learn that task.

Karen and Jim really made an effort over the next week to put into practice the plan they had developed in their therapy session. Things went well for about three days. Then one night, Ryan only slept for two hours. When they tried laying him down in his crib, he wailed inconsolably. Jim and Karen took turns with him, and with sleeping. But they were both exhausted the next morning. Karen thought she should get to sleep, because she would be home with Ryan all day, and Jim felt he should get to sleep because he had to go to work that afternoon. Neither one felt up to the task of caring for the baby, let alone doing the dishes that had become encrusted in the sink while they were dealing with Ryan. Worn out and cranky, Karen snapped at Jim about his laziness. Jim snapped back about Karen being so demanding. A full-fledged fight ensued, with lots of yelling and hurt feelings. Karen yelled that Jim didn't do enough around the house or with the baby. Jim countered with accusations that all Karen did was nag him about the housework, while he was at home, and he had started to prefer being at work.

When Karen and Jim arrived for their next session, they were still caught in this cycle of blaming and anger. They sat down on the couch, and each quickly launched into their complaints about how the other had mishandled their jobs that week. The psychologist helped them see how their mutual fatigue had led to their big blow-up, and urged them to call a truce for the next week. She pointed out how each was working hard, and each felt terribly unappreciated.

After listening to what the therapist had to say, Karen and Jim agreed to another week of trying. Each was to express appreciation for one thing done by the other every day. Karen was going to work to remind Jim about his tasks only once, and Jim was going to work to do his assigned jobs without Karen having to remind him. Karen still badly needed her breaks from Ryan, and Jim was willing to take Ryan for 30 minutes each morning, provided that Karen let him do it his way. The psychologist also stressed that Jim needed relaxation and fun, just as Karen did, and that they needed time together as a couple. Jim suggested that his mother could keep Ryan one afternoon each week so the couple might go to a movie, and he committed to working out the arrangements for this. Karen felt so touched that he was willing to put out effort for them to spend time together as a couple that she agreed to give him 20 minutes to unwind when he came home from work before she sprang on him with complaints about her day or handed him the baby to deal with.

Karen and Jim tried this new plan for a week, and found that they each felt a bit more rested and renewed. The afternoon at the movies had them each feeling almost giddy again, and much more able to handle Ryan's crying that evening. Jim sat Karen down the next evening and told her he would be much more open to her requests if they could plan the next day's schedule each day at 9 a.m. He wanted at least one day to sleep in, since he worked such late hours. He told her he would be glad to give her the same. On his day off, he agreed to let Karen go back to sleep after nursing Ryan in the morning, if he could have one other weekday morning to sleep as long as he wished. Karen was pleased that he took this initiative, and they put the plan into effect.

The extra sleep helped them both. At their next session with the psychologist, they were each feeling a bit better. When they described their week, however, it became clear that they were having some communication problems. When angered, Karen would shake her finger at Jim and speak in overgeneralizations, such as "You never do what I want," or "You always neglect the baby." When she did this, he would get sulky and withdraw, refusing to talk to her. She would keep after him until he exploded into the same types of accusations: "You never pick up your stuff either," "You always put the baby before me."

The psychologist talked with them about how helpful it can be to use "I" rather than "you" in making their needs known, such as "I am angry that you did not do as I asked right now," or "I need you to pick that up before you go to work." She also cautioned them about sticking to the complaint at hand, not dragging in every complaint from the past three years of marriage. Jim and Karen agreed to pay attention to these skills. During the following week, though, they found it hard to get rid of their old habits of communication. But when Jim took a deep breath one morning and used "I" rather than "you" when he was asking Karen to make his lunch for work, they both suddenly realized what a difference it made. A big blow-up had actually been avoided. After that, Karen wrote the doctor's suggestions on a piece of paper and taped it to the refrigerator, and Jim began to tease her gently to help her remember. When she would raise her finger to point at him accusingly, he would raise his straight up like an "I" and smile at her. This helped them each stop midstream and begin to change their habits.

By the next counseling session, it was clear that Karen and Jim were getting better at negotiating many of their differences on their own. They were communicating more clearly, and really feeling much more positively about each other. With some of the marital stress relieved, Karen realized that she still had some doubts about whether she could be a "good enough" parent. When Jim was home, she felt fairly confident, knowing he could always back her up with his wealth of infant care experience. But when Jim was working, Karen admitted that she spent a lot of time worrying about whether she was understanding Ryan's cries and giving him enough stimulation. She felt like all she did was hold Ryan or nurse him. Karen wondered if, with Ryan eight weeks of age, she should be getting more done besides baby care.

The doctor helped Karen look at what she felt she *did* do well with Ryan. Karen could identify several strengths: her loving ways, expressing lots of affection with Ryan, and her desire to do well as a parent. She decided she wanted to learn more about Ryan's development as a way to enjoy him more. The psychologist sent her to the library in search of several books about child development, and put her in touch with the "Parents as Teachers" program in her school district. This program would send out a volunteer twice a month to visit with Karen and Ryan at home. When she came, the volunteer talked with Karen about a baby's abilities at each stage of development, and gave her ideas about games to play with Ryan to both challenge his abilities and have more fun with him. When Karen had this information, she began to enjoy her time alone with Ryan much more, finding activities beyond feeding and changing to share with him. Karen continued to attend the breastfeeding support group, where she got a lot of pleasure and support comparing notes with other mothers.

Through the course of several more marital sessions, Jim and Karen continued to work on talking to each other more positively and speaking up for what each wanted rather than expecting the other to be a mind reader. It was difficult to take a deep breath and think before letting the anger and frustration come out in a hurtful manner, but they both could easily see how much happier they were with each other when they made that effort. When they had a rough week, the therapy sessions helped them see how they had not taken the time or made the effort to take care of themselves, either individually or as a couple. If Karen missed her support group meeting or her walk, she was crankier. Then it was harder to stop and think about the new skills she was learning in her marriage. If Jim had to rush right home and take on Ryan, without his 20 minutes to read the paper, he was more likely to snap at Karen. If Ryan slept little, and Jim and Karen were both tired, they had a difficult time enjoying the baby or getting the house picked up without lots of blaming going on. They had to work hard to maintain the balance of time for each other, Ryan, individual time off, the housework, and paid work. Karen found an 11-year-old neighbor to come in to the house twice a week and play with Ryan while Karen got the house cleaned up. Jim decided to designate two days a month as "honey do" days, when Karen could make him a list of home repairs or big cleaning jobs to tackle. She could relax on these two days, knowing that he would do his best to get those chores done—and this helped her ease up on her nagging.

Karen had several therapy sessions alone as well. She had quite a lot of accumulated anger about Jim distancing himself from her and Ryan in her first weeks postpartum, and decided that she needed to talk about this without Jim being there. The psychologist encouraged her to keep a notebook in which to write down her angry feelings. She also found the "silent scream" effective, where she could go into the car, roll up the window, and scream without scaring the baby or angering Jim. After 11 therapy sessions, most for the couple but some for Karen alone, Jim and Karen decided that they were feeling confident enough to continue with the changes on their own. They were communicating better, and sharing the work of parenting as they had planned to before Ryan was born. Karen was building a network of supportive friends, other parents with whom she could compare notes and share ideas. When she was able to see that many other mothers of four-month-old babies had problems similar to hers, she began to realize that a lot of it had to do with the stage, rather than her abilities. This helped her gain confidence as a parent. When Karen felt better about these things, Jim felt freer to take on extra work, contributing to the family's financial well-being. When the psychologist contacted Karen for a checkup several months later, Karen admitted that the changes still required their conscious effort. But when the effort was there, family relations ran smoothly.

Paula's Story

Paula was no stranger to postpartum depression and anxiety by the time her second baby was born. She remembered all too well the despair and consuming anxiety that had followed her first child's birth. "It began about two weeks after bringing Becky—now three years old—home from the hospital. The depression came first, with crying spells and feeling blue. Some days, I had no appetite. Becky had colic and reflux (projectile vomiting). Nothing I did would make her happy. She spent most of her waking hours crying or spitting up her food. I was totally worn out. Then the anxiety kicked in.

"Suddenly, I began worrying that if I ate anything solid, I would choke to death. I couldn't get this thought out of my mind. I wanted to stop eating altogether, but knew I needed some nourishment to have enough energy to care for my daughter. So I bought all these instant breakfasts and ready-made shakes. I would even gag on those. Still, I kept forcing myself to stay on a liquid diet, because the sight of food made me heave.

"Besides my fear of choking, I had obsessive fears about Becky's health. I stopped taking her out in the car because I was so afraid we'd have an accident. I wouldn't let anyone else feed her, for fear she would choke. I had visions of her dying from sudden infant death syndrome, and insisted to my husband that she sleep next to us in her bassinet at night. Of course, I didn't sleep much, because I was always listening to her breathing. Any slight change in the sound of it worried me. I tossed fitfully most nights, and kept her baby monitor turned on high during nap-time. My nerves didn't get a moment's rest."

By two months postpartum, Paula was thinking about killing herself. She didn't have a specific plan—she just wanted some relief for her anxiety. Feeling exhausted and hopeless, she was convinced that her life could never get any better. Too ashamed to seek treatment, she kept pushing herself to get through. As Becky's colic and reflux improved, Paula felt a little stronger. She was also fortunate to have the support of her husband and friends, who encouraged her to go on, and lent their strength whenever hers had run out. By four months postpartum, she felt that maybe she could recover after all. "I stopped thinking about harming myself. And I didn't worry nonstop any more about my daughter's health. I started getting out some, and we decided that Becky should sleep in the nursery. So I got some rest, which helped me tremendously. I'd learned my lesson about why prisoners of war are tortured with sleep deprivation! It took another six months for my eating to return to normal—at least, more like it used to be. I can't say I felt 100 percent, but most of the depression and anxiety was gone—enough for me to lead a normal life. I was thrilled."

Although Paula knew she had some chance of experiencing another postpartum reaction with a second baby, she and her husband, Brad, resolved to get help early this time. In the last trimester of her second pregnancy, her obstetrician referred her to a health-care provider who specialized in postpartum adjustment. This specialist helped Paula work out a postpartum plan to decrease the stresses she might experience. More specifically, they talked about Brad taking two weeks off after Paula delivered, to allow her more time to rest and recuperate. Brad and Paula set up a schedule for family and friends who would come over for the next four to six weeks, for a few hours every other day, to help with housework and child care. In addition, Paula began practicing relaxation techniques to reduce the anxiety if it recurred.

Paula told the counselor of her prior postpartum difficulties, and her feelings of hopelessness and despair. They agreed that it would be best for Paula not to try to "do it all" this time, and to find ways to cope with her worries and fears. The baby would *not* sleep in their room. Paula *would* allow other people to care for her child. Although she had some mild fears about choking toward the end of her pregnancy, Paula felt confident that she could avoid the postpartum problems she had before.

One week ahead of her due date, Paula gave birth to a healthy baby boy. He did not have colic or reflux, and was easy to comfort. For the first month, her postpartum recovery was problem-free. Yes, she was tired and a little blue, but she didn't have the fears and anxiety that had followed Becky's birth. About six weeks postpartum, she started weaning baby Ethan in preparation for returning to work. Boom. The anxiety over her choking hit hard. She stopped eating solid food. Sometimes she would choke on water or other fluids. Paula couldn't believe it was happening all over again.

"I thought if I did everything like we planned, I'd be okay. And it went so well at first! I really thought I was out of the woods. I felt so frustrated and disappointed. What more could I do? Why was I having those troubles? What was the matter with me? It didn't take me long to feel completely disgusted with myself. This baby was fine, so I couldn't blame my problems on him. There was something wrong with me—it was *my* fault. I was so sad, and so scared I wouldn't ever get well."

The specialist explained to her that some women develop postpartum reactions when they stop breastfeeding. In her case, this seemed to have been the likely cause. To help with reducing her anxiety and fear of choking, Paula was referred to a psychiatrist who put her on an anti-anxiety medication. She continued to work with her counselor on practicing anxiety management skills, such as relaxation. Together they worked out an eating plan to help Paula gradually reintroduce solid foods to her diet.

For the next ten months, Paula stayed in treatment until her eating returned to normal. While she felt more supported this time, she struggled with many of the feelings she experienced with her first postpartum reaction. "I was nervous that I wouldn't get better. I had worked so hard to prevent this, and it happened anyway. I was angry with myself for not having the strength to control my symptoms. I was horribly sad that I couldn't enjoy my son's infancy. But I didn't have the overwhelming despair, or thoughts of killing myself. At least that was an improvement." Shortly following Ethan's first birthday, Paula felt fully recovered. She remained in treatment anyway to practice her anxiety management skills and maintain her emotional health.

Eighteen months later, Paula was pregnant with her third child. During the first and second trimester, she met with her counselor every two weeks to monitor how she was doing. She practiced her relaxation, positive thinking, and stress management skills throughout her pregnancy. She found that these skills were helpful in her daily life, whether or not she had anxiety. For the final eight weeks, she and her counselor met weekly. She also visited with the psychiatrist who had treated her for her second postpartum episode. The two of them reviewed the steps they would take if she had another postpartum reaction. Her husband was actively involved in designing a plan to improve their postpartum adjustment, and participated in many of the counseling sessions with her. She began to see herself and her husband as a team working together to prevent postpartum difficulties. She felt that he had come a long way in understanding her distress; he seemed committed to fully supporting her, regardless of what happened.

When their third baby—a girl—was born, Paula was very worried about experiencing another postpartum reaction. As with her second child, Amy was an easy baby who slept a lot and rarely cried. The older children were delighted to have a new sister. Brad was relieved that his wife was doing well: no anxiety, no fears—just the normal upheaval that a new baby brings. But when it was time to wean Amy, Paula panicked. "I was certain my problems would start now. The first month had been so good—I knew it couldn't last. I tried not to worry about another postpartum episode. I told myself to be objective. That nothing had happened yet. I tried to be brave. I just couldn't stop the fears from coming on."

But despite her concerns and a few sleepless nights, Paula did not experience a third postpartum reaction. Days passed, then weeks, then months. Something had changed. Her treatment and planning paid off. No symptoms occurred. Finally, she could sit and rock her baby contentedly without fear or anxiety. Finally, she could enjoy the happiness that new mothers feel when they look into their child's eyes. Finally, the worst was over. A new chapter had begun.

Mary's Story

Mary and Jon were married for five years before they decided it was time to have a baby. Mary was a hospital social worker, and Jon worked as a systems analyst. Mary had grown up in a troubled family. Her parents had divorced when she was a preteenager, and she had shuttled back and forth between her parents during her teen years. Her memories of childhood were dismal: her father drank a lot, but he had been a "happy drunk." Her mother had a bad temper, and had yelled a lot, thrown things when angry, and sometimes even hit Mary and her younger sisters. When she lived with her mother, Mary was in charge of her younger sisters much of the time, having to play parent to them.

Jon was eager to have children as soon as they married, but Mary was reluctant. She felt as if she had already played parent to her siblings—why would she want to saddle herself with those responsibilities again? Family life had been so miserable for Mary during her own childhood that she convinced Jon to put off parenthood for almost four years. But when she turned 30, she decided she was ready to become a mother—and to make things different for her child than they had been for her.

Mary enjoyed a nearly picture-perfect pregnancy. She felt well, attended a prenatal exercise class at the hospital where she worked, and planned an intervention-free birth. Jon and Mary attended prepared childbirth classes together and talked with the family practitioner who would deliver their baby about their wishes for the birth. The doctor seemed supportive, and reassured them that everything would be just fine. Mary began to feel more confident about becoming a parent. Jon had what she called a "normal" family background. His parents were still together, and were very loving with each other and supportive of Jon. They treated Mary as their own daughter, and she found this love and constancy to be very comforting. Between their supportive influence, and the skills she used in her work, maybe she really could be a good parent. She still had some apprehension about this life change—about actually taking care of another person again. But Jon was so upbeat and excited, it was hard to dwell on her doubts for long.

Three weeks before Mary's due date, one of her good friends at work died of a heart attack. Mary had been close to this coworker, an older woman who had been sort of a surrogate mother for Mary. This friend had taken Mary shopping for baby clothes and furnishings, and had offered to be "babysitter on call" after Mary and Jon's baby was born. Her sudden death hit Mary very hard, leaving a painful void in Mary's life. Even though her own mother lived only 30 minutes away, Mary had learned to limit her contact with her. She never felt happy after spending time with her mother, in stark contrast to the good feelings she had always enjoyed after spending time with her friend.

When Mary went into labor, she didn't even tell Jon at first, hiding her pains from him. For Mary, a person who liked to feel in control of what was going on with her, labor was a particularly dreadful experience. Although she worked in a hospital, she hated the idea of being a patient, and having to rely on nurses to take care of her. The labor and delivery rooms were in the basement of the hospital, where it was dark and dim. So, two hours after her contractions had begun, Mary sent Jon off to work, saying she had a bad headache. Her plan was to labor at home, alone, until she couldn't stand it anymore.

She made it through the whole day, contractions still only five minutes apart, using the breathing techniques she'd learned, walking, and soaking in the shower to ease her discomfort. When Jon came home at 5:30 and saw how tired and haggard she looked, he became immediately worried and put his arms around her. This show of support and love melted her determination to "do it all alone," and she told him what she'd been through. Jon, of course, became ecstatic and wanted to call the doctor. But Mary made him hold out until 10 p.m., when the contractions were two minutes apart. They rushed to the hospital, certain that they would soon have a baby!

Arriving at the hospital, Mary and Jon were whisked into a labor room and examined by the nurse. Mary was devastated to learn that she was still only at five centimeters' dilation. As Jon went to check them in, she broke into tears, sobbing hysterically. She could not talk to the nurses, she was crying so hard. The nurse went ahead with the standard IV insertion, unable to understand Mary's protests through her tears. After that, the birth interventions snowballed, with the hospital staff ignoring Mary's wishes for the least intervention possible. Every time she complained, the staff would talk only to Jon, telling him of the necessity of the next item, whether IV, enema, fetal monitor, or medication. Mary felt totally out of control, and the staff and doctor treated her as unable to make any decisions on her own because of her hysterical crying. Finally, after an epidural and episiotomy, Mary gave birth to an 8 lb., 10 oz. baby girl. She'd had 90 minutes of pushing, and the doctor used a vacuum extractor for the final delivery. Mary and Jon spent a few minutes in the recovery room with baby Josephine, and then Mary collapsed into an exhausted sleep. She did not even wake up when the nurse brought the baby at 4 a.m. for breastfeeding, even though the nurse tapped her lightly and spoke her name.

The next day, Mary was intent on getting home right away. Since she and the baby were having no physical problems, her doctor discharged her. Back in her own bed, she was able to get some more rest, and felt as if she could at least begin to do things her way. Jon's parents came to visit, and stayed the day to help. Jon took several days off, and family and friends streamed in and out of the house, bringing food and advice, for the next three days. Mary was tired, and nursing the baby was a struggle. She seemed to have a constant headache. Everyone kept exclaiming about what a lovely baby Josey was! Mary felt more and more irritable. She missed the limelight of pregnancy. All of a sudden no one cared about how *she* felt.

About three days after Josey was born, Mary began to have very scary thoughts. She would see the block of knives on the counter, and this would trigger the thought, "I could stab the baby." Then that thought would get stuck in her head, like a broken record. "I could stab the baby, I could stab the baby, I could stab the baby"—again and again it would run through her brain. Mary was terrified. It was suddenly clear to her: this was why she should not have become a mother. All her own mother's anger and abuse were going to be repeated. Mary felt as if she was spinning out of control, and her feelings of guilt were enormous. What if she acted on these horrible thoughts? What if Jon knew about them—what would he think? What if his loving family knew? She was sure it would all end in tragedy. She thought of killing herself to save the baby. She felt certain that if she hurt the baby, she would have to kill herself. Mary was paralyzed with fear and guilt. All she could do was cry. She told no one of these thoughts; she just cried day after day. She would close herself in the bathroom at night, after Josey and Jon were asleep, and cry on the cold, hard floor, until she slept as well.

When Josey was two weeks old, Mary's younger sister, who had been her favorite, was killed in a boating accident. Mary and Jon attended the funeral, taking Josey with them. Mary cried and cried some more. Now, though, it seemed that no one worried about her crying. She was grieving her sister's death, thought Jon, and it was right that she should cry as much as she wanted. He felt absolutely helpless to comfort her. He wanted to let Mary grieve, but all she did was cry. Not knowing what else to do, Jon just let the situation go on as it was. Maybe getting back to work would help.

And getting back to work did help Mary. When Josey was seven weeks old, Mary found a sitter she trusted for the baby and went back to work part-time. She secretly felt that the sitter might be better for the baby than Mary herself. The sitter didn't have thoughts about hurting the baby, like Mary did.

The scary thoughts could be kept under control while Mary rushed around the busy hospital, tending to the concerns of others. And when Mary was home in the evening with Jon, she felt relatively safe. She could avoid looking at the knives. She stayed out of the kitchen, professing to being too tired to cook or clean up. Jon was more than willing to be accommodating, pitching in and doing much of the housework and baby care. He hoped his efforts would pay off soon, and that Mary would be "back to her old self." Mostly he just watched her, seeing how tired and overwhelmed she looked, and feeling sad that she did not seem to enjoy Josey as he did.

Mary went on like this for six months, feeling like an intense failure as a parent. She went through the motions, working and caring for Josey and the home. But she felt like she was imprisoned in a fog. Everywhere she looked, the fog was gray, and thick, and impenetrable. She did not have "the thoughts," as she called them, as frequently. But she still was plagued by guilt. How could she have had such thoughts? What sort of monster must she be? When was she going to snap, turning into an abusive parent like her mother? Sometimes she just laid Josey in her playpen and let her cry, for 30 minutes or an hour at a time, afraid to be with the baby because she might hurt her. Most nights she still stayed up late and cried after Jon and the baby were asleep. Jon had made a valiant effort to make her feel better. He had arranged for his parents to keep Josey overnight, so that he and Mary could rekindle their romantic life. Even that had been unsuccessful. After an enjoyable dinner and dancing, Mary still could not face making love. How could anyone love her, when she considered herself to be so contemptible? She shrugged off Jon's embraces and went to sleep on the sofa, crying herself to sleep again.

The next Monday Mary decided it was time to do something different. She made an appointment with her family doctor. When she got there, she told her physician about the depression she was experiencing. She explained about crying all the time, and how she had come to hate her body. She felt fat, she had blotchy skin, her feet hurt, she had frequent rashes. Mary did not tell the doctor about her disturbing thoughts. She was afraid that if she did, the doctor might call Child Welfare and take Josey away from her. In her career as a social worker, she knew the harm that could come from misunderstandings about a child's safety in the parents' home. She knew Josey was safe as long as Jon was around. The doctor gave her a prescription for *Prozac*. Mary filled it right away, and took it for a couple of weeks. She began to feel a bit better, and was not crying every day. But after about six weeks, her progress on that drug had slowed. She could not kick the feelings of guilt, and she was still crying every day. Unsure of what to do next, the doctor gave her a prescription for BuSpar, and progesterone, 100 mg. a day. Mary gave this a faithful try, feeling in her heart that probably nothing would work. She would be crabby and mean like her mother now that she was a mother, too. It was unavoidable—her "destiny."

When that new regimen made little difference in her mood, Mary's doctor referred her to a psychiatrist. This doctor prescribed norpramine, an antidepressant. Mary started to take that, but had a bad reaction. She felt light-headed and dizzy. She couldn't even get to the kitchen to call the doctor. And when she did call, the receptionist called her back, not the doctor! It turned out that Mary's doctor had gone on a six-week vacation. Mary had never met the doctor who'd be covering for him, and simply didn't have the energy to present herself and all her problems to a complete stranger.

At that point Mary just gave up. She didn't know where to turn. Jon was getting impatient. Josey was nearly one, and Mary could still not get it together. In his frustration, he began to lecture her on "showing some strength of character" and "pulling yourself up by your bootstraps." "Just smile," he would tell her, as if having the outward appearance of happiness would make her feel happy on the inside.

One day while Mary was attending to some business on the postpartum floor of the hospital, she saw a flyer about an organization called Depression After Delivery (DAD). She made a copy of the flyer, went back to the office, and called the number for more information. When the packet came in the mail three days later, Mary dove into it, searching for answers. She could not believe what she read. The descriptions of postpartum depression sounded so familiar. She had never thought of her condition as having anything to do with postpartum depression. The idea struck her that what she was going through not only had a name but might be curable! The DAD information packet contained a list of professionals nationwide who worked with postpartum depression; one of the therapists listed was local. Mary called five times, hoping to catch the doctor at his desk, before she got up the nerve to leave her name with the receptionist. The doctor called Mary back within an hour—by this time, he had gotten to know her as "that poor woman who won't leave a message"—and seemed so kind and understanding that Mary felt instant relief. Maybe her life didn't really have to be like this! She made an appointment, and went to her first therapy session without even telling Jon about it.

Mary went up in the elevator feeling a great deal of trepidation and worry. Maybe she had waited too long for this to do her any good. Josey would be one in four days. Maybe the doctor would try to take her baby away when he found out the sort of thoughts Mary had. Maybe she *was* an unfit mother. She nervously entered the room and sat down, but began to relax as the doctor went into more detail about postpartum depression, and how whatever Mary had gone through it was *not* her fault. Mary told the doctor about her urges to kill the baby and herself when Josey was young, but the doctor didn't seem in the least judgmental, or press her for more details. He reassured her that, since she was no longer having these ideas, she was probably well on her way to feeling better. Mary breathed a sigh of relief when she realized that no one was going to try to take Josey away from her. She and the doctor agreed on a plan of individual sessions for Mary, to work on how she felt about herself as a parent and a person, and to grieve the loss of her sister and her friend. They would also have some sessions with Jon and Josey to evaluate the effects of this nightmarish year on the whole family.

Jon came with Mary for the next appointment, and was much relieved to learn that she would eventually get better. The doctor told of some specific things Jon could do to help Mary, such as encouraging her. Mary needed him to acknowledge that he knew how hard it had been for her this first year of Josey's life. She needed to hear him express confidence that she would be able to get through it, with his help and the doctor's. Mary made it clear how unhelpful it was when Jon lectured or lost patience with her; he said that he was more than willing to show more compassion and sensitivity in the way he spoke to her.

Mary brought Josey with her for the next session. Even though Mary had felt depressed for most of Josey's life, it was clear to the doctor that she had bonded with the baby. Mary was gentle and affectionate with Josey, who stayed close to her mother's knee. Mary did make an effort to have some playtime with the baby every day, and Josey was one of the few people who could get her mother to smile and laugh. When the doctor reassured Mary that she'd made a terrific bond with her baby—it was obvious!—Mary began to feel like maybe she wasn't such a hopeless mother after all.

After that, Mary scheduled her sessions with the doctor on a weekly basis. She looked forward to these times, when she could finally be honest about her feelings of the past year. She liked having the doctor's concrete ideas about what she could do differently. Playing with Josey, and tucking her in at night after a satisfying bedtime routine, helped Mary feel like a competent parent—the psychologist encouraged her to stick to these routines every day. Mary learned that writing in a journal could be an effective way to get rid of some of the feelings she had simply cried about in the past. To deal with Mary's fears about Josey being taken away from her, and to literally rid herself of her scariest thoughts and feelings, the doctor suggested that she tear out and burn the pages that most upset her after she wrote them down. Mary was angry about her childhood, and having been a "parentified child," with adult responsibilities, ever since she was eight years old. She was angry about the deaths of her sister and her friend. She was angry and disappointed about her birth experience, and how Jon and the doctor hadn't stuck with the plans Mary had laid out so carefully with them in advance. Mary learned to set up specific times to cry, or worry, or pound on pillows to get her anger out. She wrote letters of goodbye to her friend and her sister, and a letter to her mother about how let down she felt, not having a mother to rely on. Mary found that feeling better was hard, for she had to actually feel many of the feelings she had been avoiding for the past year and longer. She came to accept that she could not have all good days, and that on some days she might feel like she was back to "square one."

The psychologist referred Mary to a psychiatrist, who started Mary on a higher dose of *Prozac* than she had previously tried. The medication really worked this time: Mary was ecstatic when she had her first complete night of sleep after 15 months. She felt so much better once she was sleeping. Jon even commented, "It looks like my wife is coming back." She almost felt as if this new good feeling was too good after all her time of feeling bad.

Then, about a week after she started feeling really better, Mary went to work and found a note on her desk that her supervisor wanted to meet with her. As soon as Mary had settled herself into a chair in her boss's office, the supervisor began to gently explain how the department had had numerous complaints about Mary's interactions with patients and their families during this past year.

Mary was devastated. All this time, she had believed that she was doing a good job at work, despite her troubles at home and her depression. Now she felt like a total failure. The supervisor had noticed that Mary was feeling better, and thought that she would be ready to handle some negative feedback about her job performance. Mary went into a tailspin. Here her "fog" had been evident to all those around her, while she thought she was doing fine. She quickly slipped back into the depression she had just begun conquering, crying almost nonstop. The following week she confided to her therapist that she had been saving up her medication and planned to kill herself. When the psychologist, much concerned, began to discuss the need to put Mary in the hospital, to protect her from killing herself or hurting anyone else, Mary quit talking. She suddenly became very withdrawn, rocking in her chair and hugging her knees tightly. The therapist called Jon, and the psychiatrist, and they made arrangements to hospitalize Mary.

In the hospital, Mary remained withdrawn for several days. With the addition of lithium to her medication, and the support of the hospital staff, her psychologist, and Jon and his family, Mary was feeling much better after two weeks' time. She stayed in the hospital for 21 days in all, and continued her individual therapy with her psychologist. Mary focused over the next couple of months on the issues surrounding Josey's infancy and Mary's role as a mother. She talked to her own mother about how she never complimented Mary. Her mother was able to take this to heart, and began to tell Mary what a great job she was doing with Josey. Mary learned to make a list of positive things she had accomplished each day, and to review the list at the end of the day. She found it worked best to note one positive thing about her work, one about her parenting, and one about another quality she liked in herself. Once she felt more on track with these issues, Mary felt ready to address her anger and frustration about her childbirth experience and the mess she felt her body was in. She began to take an exercise class on a regular basis. She wrote out her birth story, and saw how she had really done as well as she could within the context of a tough, unsupported experience. She brought Jon in for another therapy session, to tell him of her anger about how he didn't stick to the birth plan they'd made together. He held his ground, saying that he had trusted the medical personnel; but he was really sorry to have caused her additional pain. Mary felt better just knowing that he now understood how she'd felt betrayed and abandoned by him. Mary spent a lot of time exploring stress management, and ways she might handle her stressful job and family situation by taking more time for herself, even in five-minute pieces throughout the day.

By the time Josey was 18 months old, Mary was feeling almost like her old self again, only better. And then she was devastated to find herself pregnant.

Even though she was feeling so much better, and had learned a great deal about how to cope, Mary was terrified that she would go through the same sort of nightmare again if she had another baby. Her psychologist worked to reassure her. But Mary became quite depressed again, had difficulty sleeping, and cried a great deal.

To make things worse, she had to discontinue her medication because of the pregnancy. The first trimester was pretty rough, both physically and emotionally. Mary "rode it out" with the support of her therapist, Jon, and two good friends. By the second trimester, she was feeling better physically and could reestablish her exercise routine. With the more stable hormones of this time period, Mary was sleeping better, too. She began to plan for this new baby's arrival, with great care paid to what she could do to avoid the depression and obsessive thoughts. Together, Mary and Jon took a prepared childbirth class based on the Bradley method. They drew up a birth plan in consultation with Mary's family practitioner, had him sign it, and made sure that it was put into Mary's chart. That way, even if another doctor attended her birth, all of Mary and Jon's stipulations would have to be followed. Mary hoped to be able to have more control over her birth experience this time, and to avoid the feelings of anger and disappointment she had felt with Josey's birth. With her psychologist's help, she looked into the use of progesterone to prevent postpartum depression. Jon's family volunteered to be on hand to care for the house and Josey, and plans were made to have Jon and his mother alternate with the new baby's night feedings for the first week so that Mary could get enough sleep.

Baby Ellen joined her sister Josey after a ten-hour labor and completely unmedicated birth. Mary and Jon were ecstatic. They had worked well as a team this time, and had been able to avoid all unnecessary medical intervention, even using the birthing room at the hospital. Tired but satisfied, they left the hospital when Ellen was six hours old. Mary wanted to leave as soon as possible and recuperate at home.

All went well for about three days. Then Mary was horrified to find that she was again having thoughts about hurting her baby. She couldn't stop thinking about stabbing her. Mary felt destroyed. All her careful planning couldn't prevent the nightmare from coming again. As she felt the fog settle over her, Mary became tearful and withdrawn. She was just able to muster the energy to call her psychologist and cry for help.

Extremely concerned, the psychologist checked with a psychiatrist about the proper dose for the progesterone Mary was taking. It turned out that Mary's family practitioner had prescribed only one-fourth of the dosage needed. After a call from Mary's therapist, the doctor agreed to up the dose. Meanwhile, Mary met with Jon and the psychologist. Mary had never told Jon about her obsessive thoughts about hurting Josey, or that they'd been at the heart of Mary's depression. He was shocked at first. The therapist explained that such thoughts are caused by changing brain chemistry related to the sudden drop in female hormones postpartum. He emphasized that the thoughts weren't Mary's fault, and were not even related to Mary's early family history. This set Jon's mind somewhat at ease. Not trusting the progesterone by itself now, Mary resumed taking *Prozac* as well, which was likely to diminish her obsessive thoughts.

Within three days on the larger dose of progesterone plus *Prozac*, Mary was feeling well again. The thoughts were almost completely gone.

When she had an occasional thought about hurting the baby, she would say to herself, "This is just a thought. I'm not going to act on it, and it says nothing about me as a parent or a person."

Mary felt like a "normal person" after that. She was enjoying baby Ellen much more than she had ever been able to enjoy Josey. This made her feel sad for the loss of Josey's infancy, and she had to use her journaling and grieving skills to let go of that sadness, too. She found she could balance almost everything she wanted to do if she managed to break everything down into small steps and interim goals. She made lists for every day of the week, and reviewed them by herself and with Jon to make sure her goals were reasonable. Always good at getting organized, Mary quickly got Josey and Ellen on schedules, so she could have ten minutes here and there to herself every day for reading or journaling. When Jon proposed a weekend without the baby and Josey, Mary was delighted to find herself looking forward to that time alone. She still hated the extra pounds she was stuck with from her two pregnancies, but tried to believe that Jon found her attractive, even if she didn't like the way she looked right now. She reminded herself that she could lose the extra weight when she started exercising again. And she was going to give herself a reasonable amount of time to do that and to be gentle and kind with herself throughout her postpartum recovery—and maybe even for the rest of her life.

9

Before the Storm:
Prenatal Planning

The Short Version
(If You're Pressed For Time)

It is clear that much can be done to prevent and/or at least diminish postpartum problems through sound preconceptual and prenatal planning. This is true for all women, and especially for those who are at high risk for a postpartum reaction. If you have experienced a prior postpartum episode and are pregnant now, you should read this chapter. Don't underestimate the importance of prenatal preparation as a means to improve your chances for a healthy postpartum adjustment.

Prenatal Planning

There are really two parts to prenatal planning: preparing for motherhood before you actually become pregnant, and planning for your postpartum adjustment once you are pregnant. Just as you may be eating right and exercising to insure a healthy conception, it is equally important to assess your emotional readiness. First, consider if you feel psychologically ready to become pregnant, and to undertake the emotional challenges of pregnancy and motherhood. Next, evaluate whether you and your partner are ready for this step. If you need to work on your individual preparedness, or your relationship, take care of this now, prior to pregnancy.

Once you become pregnant, resolve any significant individual or relationship problems early on. Seek professional help if necessary. Whatever your situation, plan for your postpartum adjustment. Decide how you and your partner will divide child-care and household responsibilities. Rough out a nighttime feeding schedule. Review what your priorities will be for the first two to three months postpartum, and who will assist you in meeting your goals. Be certain to spend time enjoying your partner's company before your child's birth.

Reducing Your Risk

If you have a history of postpartum problems, or there's some other factor that increases your risk, plan carefully for postpartum changes. Deal with previous postpartum difficulties that have persisted. Address personal and relationship problems immediately. Design a postpartum plan that will eliminate or reduce potential difficulties. Finally, select a physician and team of health-care providers who know how to treat postpartum reactions, and develop a contingency plan with them.

Motherhood Revisited

As a society, it is critical that we embrace a new view of motherhood that recognizes the postpartum period as a time of tremendous challenge and change. Motherhood is a learning process, not something that happens overnight. There is no single right way to be a mom: every woman should be supported in creating her own style of mothering. With this change in attitude, new moms may begin to see themselves in a kinder, more forgiving light; to perceive their differences as strengths, and to see their mistakes as an opportunity to learn something new.

Exercise
Two Minutes for Yourself

Do this exercise if you're pregnant. Sit in a comfortable chair with your feet up, or sit cross-legged on the floor—whatever feels right for you. Place your hands lightly over your belly and close your eyes. Think about the life inside you: your baby is completely part of you now. Your body knows exactly what to do to keep the baby comfortable, nourished, and clean. Your body is doing a fantastic job, and it's doing it just right.

Try to sense the baby through your hands—it doesn't matter if you're nine months pregnant and due any day now, or if you've just found out you're pregnant. Just touch lightly and think about the life inside you. When your baby is born, everything will be much more complicated, and you won't always know what to do. Now your body knows exactly what to do, and does it perfectly, without you even having to think about it. Take a deep breath and tell yourself that it won't be like this after the baby's umbilical cord is cut and you become two creatures instead of one. Once you're separated, the baby will have to learn how to tell you what he or she needs, and you'll have to learn to understand. Unless you've spent a lot of time around newborn babies, it will be as difficult as learning a foreign language. Take another deep breath. Accept the prospect of this challenge. You're going to make mistakes—this is an inevitable part of the learning process.

Put your energy in your hands again. Your baby will love you. You are everything to your baby—you are life itself. Give love to your child and your child will give you love in return. This is the one thing you can know with certainty. The rest is unknowable.

Take another deep breath. You will not be able to control everything about your child's life—in fact, you will be able to control very little, and you'll have less and less control as your child grows up. Tell yourself that this is okay. This is the way of the world. When you focus on the things you can change, you'll find that most of them are inside you. You can grow in your knowledge and in your love. You can never learn to be a perfect mother, because such a being doesn't exist. What you can learn to be is good enough.

Now take your hands off your belly and pat yourself on the back.

9

Before the Storm:
Prenatal Planning

Long before your baby was born, you probably thought about becoming a mom, and what your baby would be like. You may have timed your pregnancy to coincide with a slow period at work, or a certain time of year. You may have adjusted your diet and exercise routine to prepare for pregnancy and childbirth. You may have imagined yourself holding your baby, and singing a special lullaby. You may have planned your child's room, and mentally selected the outfit you wanted your newborn to wear home from the hospital. In many ways, you are likely to have planned the details of your baby's arrival well ahead of time.

But few women make plans for their own care as they envision a life for their baby. Although there is no way you can fully prepare yourself for the tremendous physical, emotional, and relationship changes that occur postpartum, there are things you can do ahead of time to ease your transition to motherhood. Following the guidelines in this chapter may smooth your postpartum adjustment and lower your chances of a postpartum reaction. Even before you become pregnant, there are steps you can take to decrease your likelihood of experiencing postpartum problems. During pregnancy, there is much you can do. If you are at high risk for postpartum difficulties according to the Risk Profile Questionnaire in Chapter 3, you will want to pay particular attention to the prenatal recommendations in this chapter. Most women who are at high risk can significantly reduce their chances of having a postpartum reaction through prenatal planning and intervention. An ounce of prevention is once again truly worth a pound of cure.

Finally, we hope in this chapter (and throughout this book) to promote a new view of motherhood that recognizes the enormous physical, psychological, and relationship changes that come with having a child. The more society accepts that the transition to motherhood can present women with tremendous challenges as well as rewards, the more freedom women will feel to acknowledge without shame any difficulties they encounter, and to seek out the help they need.

So, You Want to Have a Baby— Prepregnancy Planning

Many women think about having a baby well in advance of becoming pregnant. If you are thinking about getting pregnant, or actively trying, now is an excellent time to start planning for your postpartum adjustment. Although this may sound like jumping the gun, it isn't. The idea of planning before pregnancy—or "preconceptual planning"—is not a new one. For years, childbirth specialists have been discussing the importance of good preconceptual physical health to insure a healthy pregnancy. In fact, many women are following this advice by establishing healthy diet and exercise habits prior to conception.

If you're trying to get pregnant, you might want to start taking prenatal vitamins before the fact (consult your doctor or nutritionist). But vitamin supplements can't replace a healthy diet. Go for high-fiber, low-fat foods, including lots of fresh fruits and vegetables, and low-fat sources of protein in your diet. Exercise three times a week to keep your body strong and fit. The better physical shape you're in, the better able you'll be to deal with the physical stresses of pregnancy and childbirth. Exercise will also enhance your emotional well-being. Cultivate good sleeping habits, and learn to rest when you feel physically or emotionally tired. Learn to recognize your own warning signs of fatigue, and learn to honor them by taking a break to replenish yourself. Putting these steps into practice now will increase your chances of a healthy pregnancy. Maintaining them after your baby is born will improve your postpartum adjustment, and decrease your risk for postpartum problems.

Psychological Readiness

One aspect of preconceptual planning that is often neglected is how to prepare yourself emotionally for becoming pregnant. This may involve assessing your psychological readiness for having a baby, and addressing past and present emotional problems that may still be bothering you. Psychological readiness refers to how prepared you feel and how capable of coping with a baby. To sort this out, ask yourself the following questions:

- How ready am I to focus my attention on a new baby, and to put my own needs aside when I have to? (This does not mean neglecting yourself, but attending to your child's immediate needs first.)
- Do I feel "grown up" enough to care for another person's total well-being?
- How responsible am I in other areas of my life, and where do I fall short? (Keep in mind that wanting a baby is different from dealing with the daily responsibilities of having a newborn.)
- How much in order are other areas of my life, including work and my partnership or marriage?
- What traits or skills do I have that will benefit me as a parent?
- What knowledge or skills would I do well to strengthen?
- Do I have any serious shortcomings that might interfere with my ability to be a caring and responsible parent? If so, what are they, and what can I do about them?
- Does this seem like the right time in my life to become a mom? (Although no time is perfect, some times are certainly more promising than others.)

Once you've thought about the answers to these questions, consider any past and/or current psychological difficulties that may affect your postpartum adjustment. For example, if you've had problems with responsibility before, and feel that you haven't worked this out, get help *before* you decide to get pregnant (or get help now if you're already pregnant). Past episodes of depression or anxiety are risk factors for the postpartum period (review the psychological risk factors described in Chapter 3). If you've had professional help and/or medication for these problems, make sure that your OB is fully aware of this aspect of your medical history. Get in touch with your counselor again to talk about the particular stresses associated with pregnancy and postpartum adjustment, and to make a plan for aggressively dealing with problems if they arise. If your counselor seems ignorant about postpartum adjustment issues, find another one (see Chapter 7). Maybe you didn't have a "good enough" relationship with your own mom, and are concerned about how this will affect your parenting. If you were abused or neglected as a child, and haven't yet dealt with these highly charged emotional issues, find a way to deal with them now, before you have a child of your own. In general, attend to any emotional issues that have the potential to interfere with your parenting and postpartum adjustment. You have time to attend to these issues now: you won't have any time for them after your baby is born. Doing something now about potential problems may spare you, your partner, and your baby a great deal of emotional pain.

Relationship Readiness

Besides feeling ready yourself to undertake the changes that accompany childbirth, you will want to look at how ready you and your partner are to become parents. This may include discussing what each of you thinks it will be like to have a child, and how you imagine parenthood will affect you as a couple. Even if this isn't your first child, discussing your expectations about how another child will affect your relationship and your family can still be worthwhile. Start talking now about how you will share the child-care and household responsibilities once your baby is born. This is a much better time for any major disagreements or minor problems to be resolved than when you are leaving the hospital with the baby in your arms.

Most importantly, if you are experiencing problems in your relationship with your partner, now is the time to work things out. Even the healthiest couples have conflicts and problems from time to time. But if problems are characteristic of your relationship, and often result in serious conflicts or painful emotions, you should probably get help together as a couple before having a child. Another warning flag is if you and your partner rarely solve any of your problems, and are unable to compromise with each other. If there is a generally negative feeling between the two of you, chances are that you're not communicating very well. Get professional help to help you change your relationship (or don't have a baby until you're in a better relationship).

Many minor relationship difficulties can be resolved simply by talking openly about them with your partner. Partners, both in business and in love, often get into trouble with each other because they don't know how to communicate effectively. Start by talking with your partner about what is bothering you, and see if the two of you can work it out. If not, a professional helper may be able to mediate your differences, or give each of you a fresh perspective. Whatever approach you decide to take, straighten out your relationship before you get pregnant. Having a baby has rarely saved a troubled relationship, and usually makes things much, much worse.

So, You Just Found Out You're Pregnant— Prenatal Planning

Just as there are steps you can take after your baby arrives to have a healthier postpartum adjustment (see Chapter 4), there are definite steps you can take during your pregnancy to improve your response to post-partum changes. These steps will differ as you move through various phases of your pregnancy, and may need to be adjusted to fit your unique circumstances. Like all the recommendations in this book, these guidelines are not set in stone, nor should you use them as a measuring rod. Every woman—and every pregnancy—is different. Your goal in taking these steps during your pregnancy is to assume an active role in programming a smoother postpartum adjustment for yourself. As you've learned by now if you've read most of the rest of this book, expectations play a crucial role in the outcome of every woman's adjustment to motherhood. The more conscious you are about these expectations, and the more you're able to bring them into line with reality, the better chance you have of a relatively easy postpartum adjustment.

The First Trimester

Pregnancy itself results in tremendous physical and hormonal changes. If you haven't done so already, the first trimester is a good time to develop a plan for caring for your physical health during the rest of your pregnancy. This plan should include a balanced diet, exercising on a regular basis (with your doctor's approval), and getting adequate rest and sleep. Especially in the first trimester, when your body's chemical balance is changing so rapidly, you want to develop some habits of flexibility so that you can adapt to your changing physical needs and "roll with the punches" if unexpected problems arise. In the past ten years, it has become increasingly clear that our physical health affects our emotional health: it's difficult to be healthy physically without being healthy emotionally, and vice versa. By following a sound health plan throughout your pregnancy, you may be able to lower your risk of postpartum adjustment problems. Get good prenatal care, give up any unhealthy habits now, and get professional help if you can't give them up on your own.

The first trimester is also a good time to take stock of any current personal or relationship difficulties that could grow into bigger problems. First, ask yourself if you are having any problems that need to be addressed. Then take a long, hard look at your relationship. Don't ignore or shy away from issues that concern you. You still have seven or eight months in which to make changes. Investing the time now can save you pain and disappointment later.

Even if your relationship seems to be in good shape, both you and your partner may want to assess your current ability to handle stress. Having a newborn can upset the whole balance of a relationship, and will increase your stress as a couple by an order of magnitude. What do you do to relax now, and how successful are you at taking time out for yourself? If you don't have relaxation skills now, acquire them, so that they'll be available to you when your baby arrives. We list some of our favorite books on stress reduction in the Resources Section; many others are available as well. Experiment to see which techniques suit you best. Then practice relaxation a few times a week until you're really good at it. Deep breathing, progressive muscle relaxation, and meditation are three stress-reduction techniques of proven merit. They can be used alone or in combination, and will be valuable resources to you in the postpartum period, when you will be under a lot of stress and may be getting less sleep than you need.

Try to learn to take time out for yourself. Set aside a specified period during the week that is "your time," and devote it to doing whatever you want to, without interruptions. You can practice taking as little as one half-hour to yourself two or three times a week. Developing a healthy respect for your needs for rest and relaxation—and teaching others in your life to respect these needs—may improve your postpartum adjustment, and decrease your chances of a postpartum reaction.

The Second Trimester

Unlike the first trimester, with its nausea and attendant fatigue, the second trimester is a time of physical and emotional well-being for many pregnant women. If you *are* feeling well during this time, finish up as much as you can of the physical preparations related to your baby's arrival. Get the baby's room ready. Complete any other household projects that will bug you if they're not done by the time the baby is born. Don't start any new projects now. Tie up loose ends at work. Assemble your baby's wardrobe and baby-care products you'll need for the first few months. Make sure you have some loose comfortable clothes you'll be able to wear. If you're really energetic, start filling your freezer with home-cooked meals—you'll be grateful later that you did so.

While you are feeling good and energized, you may want to take a vacation or pursue some other fun activities. Don't spend all your time getting ready for your baby. You need to take time to enjoy yourself, and to spend time with your partner. Do the fun things you want to *before* your baby is born. Go to the movies. Go out to restaurants. Do all the things that will be difficult or impossible later, at least for a while.

Try to strike a balance between work and pleasure. If you take good care of yourself now, you are less likely to feel angry and resentful after your baby arrives, when leisure time will be scarce. Keep your emotional pitcher full so you will have more to give later without feeling emotionally drained.

With your abdomen expanding, and your baby noticeably moving around, the reality of having this child may be setting in. This makes the second trimester an opportune time to start addressing some of the changes that your baby's birth will bring. If you have other children, talk to them about concerns they may have about the arrival of a new brother or sister. Older children may benefit from a sibling class if one is offered by your local hospital. Younger children who don't fully understand what is going on, or are unable to verbally express themselves, may benefit from picture books about new babies and the siblings who must deal with them.

Besides preparing your children, you will probably want to continue reviewing with your partner how you plan to divide child-care and household chores. Make sure that your expectations in this area are the same. The first weeks postpartum are a rotten time to discover major differences. Negotiate any differences while you still have time. Putting off your discussions until the last minute, or until after the fact, is only likely to increase conflict, and will intensify the relationship strain that normally accompanies childbirth.

If you are planning to have a part- or full-time child-care provider other than you or your partner, start investigating your options now. It may take a while to find a provider or a facility you like, and many child-care facilities have waiting lists.

As a general rule, it's best to do what you can in advance of giving birth. This will give you less to worry about later, and lower your risk of postpartum problems. Try to bear in mind, though, that no matter how well you plan, it's impossible to account for a whole host of uncontrollable and unpredictable factors. You can't control whether you'll be doomed to bed rest for the last third of your pregnancy. You can't predict what kind of labor and delivery you'll have, and whether you'll need a Caesarian. You can't control what kind of baby you'll have: and you'll have to take the luck of the draw, whether that means a baby who's placid and sleepy or wildly colicky. Do what you can about the things that *are* controllable; and remain flexible about the rest.

The Third Trimester

As you enter your third trimester, take advantage of the energy you have to finalize your labor and delivery plans. If you haven't yet selected a hospital or place where you want to deliver, figure this out. Review options regarding labor and delivery with your health-care provider. You and your partner can write up a birth plan, have it approved by your doctor, and put into your medical chart. That's one way of insisting that things go as much your way as possible during your labor and delivery.

Participate in a Lamaze or other prepared childbirth class. These classes can be enormously helpful in reviewing the labor and delivery process, and will provide you with many coping techniques for the stresses of labor.

If this is your first baby, squeeze in all the time you can to enjoy being with your partner. Toward the end of this trimester, you may be more physically fatigued and less enthusiastic about going out and having fun. If you have other children, make time to do things you enjoy with them. Let them plan a special day with you. Keep sharing lots of hugs and kisses. Remind them that although things will change with their new brother or sister's birth, they are still special and important to you.

During your third trimester, set time aside to develop a postpartum plan following the guidelines discussed in Chapter 4.

Finally, acquaint yourself with the warning signs of postpartum depression, anxiety, and psychosis. Refer back to Chapter 2 for a complete list of symptoms, and checklists for particular problems. Remember that if your symptoms last beyond four weeks, and if they get worse instead of better, you probably have postpartum depression and/or anxiety. Make a plan now about what you will do if such problems develop. Speak with your doctor or health-care providers about how you want them to assist you or ask them for their ideas. Review your plan with your partner. Although postpartum difficulties are not fully avoidable, being prepared and taking action may stop them from getting out of control.

Women at High Risk: Preventing Future Problems

Because of biology, psychology, and relationship factors, some women will be more likely than others to experience postpartum problems. You may have been drawn to this book because you've experienced postpartum problems in the past, or are experiencing them now. A past postpartum reaction increases your risk of another one dramatically, doubling your chances. Refer back to Chapter 3 for details about other risk factors. Look at these and decide whether your risk for postpartum problems is high, medium, or low. If you fall into the high or medium categories, follow the recommendations below.

Attending to a previous postpartum reaction.   First, deal with any previous postpartum difficulties that have persisted. If you think you still have symptoms of depression or anxiety that have lasted since your last baby's birth, seek professional help. Without treatment, you may not be able to fully recover from an earlier postpartum reaction. Many women suffer through one or more initial episodes of postpartum depression or anxiety before getting help.

In a support group meeting, Audrey painfully related the postpartum depression she had with her two children. Now pregnant with another child, she was trying to prevent a third postpartum episode. "I guess it wasn't so bad with my first baby—I cried off and on for the first few months, and couldn't eat or sleep much. But, gradually, it went away. My second daughter's birth was a total nightmare. I felt bad for over a year. I would cry and shake, and was frightened about leaving my house. I didn't want to have anything to do with my daughter. I regretted having another baby, and felt guilty for feeling this way. I shut myself off from my husband and friends. Nothing made me happy. I thought it would be a relief to die."

Even if you no longer have symptoms, you may need to deal with the feelings triggered by an earlier postpartum reaction. You may still feel angry, sad, guilty, or disappointed about what happened to you. Despite how much you may have tried to push these feelings aside, they may be haunting you. Very often, women who have postpartum difficulties feel a deep sense of loss over their postpartum experiences. After all, having a baby is supposed to be one of the happiest times in your life. If this turns out not to be true for you, the disappointment can be tremendous. Allowing yourself to grieve your lost dreams can be healing. Working on this now will help prevent further problems later.

Marie was a 32-year-old mother of one who sought counseling during her second pregnancy. She had suffered miserably through the first year following her daughter's birth with symptoms of mania and depression. She admitted that she wasn't cured, and couldn't bear to go through that kind of pain again. In counseling, she frequently talked about feelings she had not addressed from her first postpartum experience.

"I knew I wasn't over it, and that there were things I had to talk about. I carried a lot of guilt with me for not being a better mom to my daughter from the time she was born. But, mostly, I felt sad about how much I'd missed out on. I couldn't recall my daughter's infancy. I couldn't remember holding her when I brought her home from the hospital. So much loss—it just went on and on. My counselor told me it was normal to feel this way, and encouraged me to grieve. She gave me a chance to let my feelings out. By the time of my second daughter's birth, I felt that I had really put what happened with my first daughter behind me. I don't know what things would have been like if I hadn't gone for help."

Adjusting Your Expectations, Taking Care of Yourself, Reducing Stress. If you are at high risk, take stock of other problems that may increase your chances of postpartum difficulties. For example, if you know you tend to have high expectations of yourself, work on this. Practice lowering your expectations about being the "perfect" career woman, wife, or mother. Deliberately do less than what you think is adequate. See what response you get from yourself and others. Check how this makes you feel. Practice doing less, or doing less well, on a weekly or daily basis. If you can't do this on your own, and you feel as if your expectations are controlling you, consult a professional helper. Remind yourself that changing high-risk habits before your baby's birth will increase your chances of a healthy postpartum adjustment.

Besides changing high-risk habits, work on your ability to take care of yourself. Practice making time to do what *you* want to do. Learn to say no. Put your name on your priority list. Set 30 minutes aside each day during which no one is allowed to interrupt you. Let your partner cook dinner. Turn your phone off. Delegate responsibilities to other family members. The choices are limitless. But whatever you choose, don't back down because other things seem more pressing. Keep telling yourself, "I count. I am important. I will treat myself with care."

Try to keep lifestyle stress to a minimum. Do not buy a new house or change jobs, unless you have no other choice. That goes for your partner, too. Make your current residence more pleasing, or attend to what you like about your current job. While you won't be able to totally eliminate stress from your life, there are still some elements you can control. If you're accustomed to leading a fast-paced life, slow down. Learn to take breaks. Plan a day to do absolutely nothing. Start reducing your "have to" list. Spend 20 minutes a day meditating and clearing your mind. Resist the urge to do more. Avoid any other projects or commitments during your last trimester or your first six months postpartum. A newborn baby is challenging enough for anyone.

Building Healthier Relationships

If you are at high risk for postpartum problems, address any problems with your partner as soon as possible. Relationship stress is a primary cause of postpartum difficulties. Make certain that you and your partner work out major differences before your child's birth. This doesn't mean that you have to agree 100 percent—just so long as you agree enough to allow you to cooperate as partners and parents. If you don't communicate well, read a book on couples communication or attend a class. Professional help is another option. Effective communication is critical to your success both as partners and parents. Preserve your relationship by spending time together and don't let other responsibilities interfere with your time. Too many couples drift apart after having children.

Be sure that you have a strong social support system. Having other people to depend on for emotional and practical support will reduce your stress. Speak with family and friends about how they can help you postpartum. If you lack social support, look for ways to increase it. Try to meet other women and couples who are expecting. Join a pregnancy exercise class or prenatal education class: many hospitals sponsor these. Become active in community or religious organizations. Many such organizations are family-centered and will welcome your participation. Join a women's group. Spend more time with acquaintances from work, or in your neighborhood. Renew old friendships. Strengthen your support system however you can, because you'll desperately need it to be in place when your baby is born.

Designing a Postpartum Plan to Reduce Your Risk of Adjustment Problems

Finally, you and your health-care providers need to carefully prepare a postpartum plan of action. Your plan should include measures to lower your chances of a postpartum reaction, and contingency plans to carry out if a postpartum reaction occurs.

To decrease your odds of postpartum problems, follow the general guidelines presented in this chapter and Chapter 4. Think about what your particular risk factors may be, and how you can mitigate them. If you believe that your difficulties in the past were mostly due to physical changes, discuss this with your doctor or midwife. He or she may have specific recommendations about what to do. For example, some women who have had a previous postpartum episode choose to receive progesterone shots within 24 hours after delivery, and for several weeks thereafter. This kind of preventive treatment may be something that you and your health-care provider want to consider. Discuss all your options, and then base your decisions on your best judgment of the situation.

If you believe that psychological factors strongly contributed to your postpartum difficulties, consider adding a mental-health practitioner to your prenatal and postpartum health-care team. Ask your doctor or midwife to suggest someone. Get a referral through a local postpartum support group or the hospital where you plan to deliver. Find out if there is a mental health provider in your community who specializes in postpartum reactions. Read or review Chapter 7 if you decide to seek professional help.

It's critical to decide in advance the role to be played by each of your health-care providers if you experience a postpartum reaction. The best way to prevent postpartum difficulties from getting out of hand is to take quick and effective action.

Dominique was a 35-year-old mother of one who experienced postpartum depression after the birth of her first child. After suffering through six months of depression, she sought treatment. Gradually, her symptoms diminished, but her self-esteem was very low; she planned never to get pregnant again. "I couldn't bear the thought of going through another depression. I had felt so hopeless, and so inadequate. It was like a nightmare that wouldn't end."

Years later, Dominique changed her mind about having another child. During her third trimester, she and her husband met with the psychologist who had previously treated her, and together all three of them designed a postpartum plan. This included what Dominique and her husband planned to do to decrease postpartum stress. She planned to have her mom and dad come over daily the first month, and two or three times a week the second month, if Dominique was doing well. She decided not to breastfeed, so that she could get more sleep. She and her husband identified areas, such as housework, where they'd agree to cut back and lower their standards. Their therapist went over the warning signs of postpartum depression with Dominique and her husband. Before her due date, Dominique met with the psychiatrist who would prescribe medicine for her if she needed it.

The first couple of weeks postpartum went fine. But by the end of the first month, Dominique was experiencing symptoms of depression. Instead of waiting, she went on medication immediately, and met weekly with her psychologist, who monitored her progress. They planned from week to week what needed to be done. "I felt horrible that it was starting all over again," said Dominique later. "I was afraid of how depressed I would become. I kept thinking I had made a mistake to have another baby. But it never got that bad the second time. Sure, it was hard. But I know that it would have been much worse if I hadn't lined up the help I needed ahead of time."

Although prenatal planning can never totally eliminate your risk of postpartum difficulties, it can significantly lower it. Any investment of time and energy to this end will be more than worthwhile.

Changing Attitudes About Motherhood

The way in which motherhood is romanticized in our culture fosters many unrealistic expectations, which women often strive to meet but fail to achieve. Rather than rejecting society's expectations as unrealistic, women tend to see themselves as the problem. One mother told us, "When I thought of becoming a mother, I pictured myself singing to my baby, and walking her in her buggy—happy all the time, thoroughly enjoying being a mom. And when that didn't happen, I blamed myself. I would look at my daughter, and feel certain that someone else could take better care of her than I could. That someone else would know what to do. I kept thinking that maybe I didn't deserve to have this baby, and yet all my life I had wanted to be a mom. What was wrong with me?"

To deal with postpartum problems, and perhaps even to prevent them, society must embrace a new view of motherhood, one that recognizes the period following childbirth as a time of tremendous physical, emotional, and interpersonal upheaval. Although having a child can be joyful in many ways, it also involves enormous challenge and change. Adopting a more balanced view of motherhood may help women to stop blaming themselves for their struggles postpartum. If the period following childbirth is expected to be difficult, women may see their problems as part of a normal adjustment process, not as a personal shortcoming. They may feel more comfortable asking for assistance from family and friends, and to speak up when problems occur rather than suffering in silence. A change in society's attitude may give women permission to be more loving and gentle toward themselves as they learn to be moms, and to appreciate their strength to carry on.

A second social belief that needs to change is the assumption that mother-knowledge somehow occurs spontaneously when a woman gives birth. Although mothering is biologically programmed to a minor extent, it is mostly a learning process. Just as it takes time and practice to become an accomplished musician, it takes time and practice to learn to be a great mom. Why doesn't society reinforce this message? Women are taught to believe that they are somehow supposed to know what to do—from changing diapers to choosing preschools—from the moment their child is born. The pressure of this expectation can be crushing. How can you ask for help about something you "should" already know? And what if someone else catches you making a mistake? Your ignorance or uncertainty then becomes an occasion for shame—just one more reason to feel bad about yourself.

When society acknowledges that mothering is a learning process, many new options will arise. Women can be more patient with themselves, because everyone knows that learning a new skill takes time. Mistakes can become opportunities to learn something new, rather than ammunition for self-contempt. Less experienced moms may be more likely to get assistance and advice from the best teachers of all: moms who have been through it all before. Shame and blame will diminish for what you don't know. *Learning*, instead of *knowing*, will be the operative word.

Finally, there is the Supermom myth to dispose of. This myth implies that there is some single, right way to be a good mom. It suggests that one style of mothering is better than all others. And that anyone who falls short of this ideal is made of inferior goods. The image of Supermom has changed as often as hemlines. These days, Supermom is loving but firm. She listens, then acts. She's in control of her feelings. Supermom of the '90s is supportive but encourages independence. She's informed and active, attentive to her children's needs. She's attentive to her own needs as well. She's involved, soft, strong, capable, and mature. She's an emotional giant. She always knows the right thing to do, and does it all perfectly. Whether she stays at home or works outside her home, her life is totally in order. She never misses a beat. She is the standard of success. Hers is the image many women compare themselves to. No wonder they feel so bad!

Telling yourself that you have to be Supermom is like telling yourself that you need to look like a high-fashion model: it's possible, given the right natural endowments, but it's not something that very many people can do. And it's ridiculous and self-destructive to hold yourself to such impossibly high standards. Society must let go of the notion that there is only one way to be a good mom. Motherhood is an extremely complicated role—so complex, in fact, that perfection and always being right are simply impossible. Every mother makes mistakes, because mothers are only human.

There are many useful and loving approaches to motherhood. It is up to each woman to develop her own style, and to follow her heart. When society promotes diversity, there will be no shame in not conforming to one particular view of the ideal. Women will be able to feel self-esteem and self-acceptance *because* they are different, if their difference springs from an individual vision of what is right and good. We can then let go of the contempt and self-hatred we inflict on ourselves when we fall short of some unattainable ideal.

10

Putting It All Together

Just from reading this book, you may already be feeling better. We hope so. You may have learned the name for what you're experiencing, whether this is postpartum depression, postpartum anxiety, or a postpartum thought disorder. It's to be hoped that you feel reassured: you're not crazy or weak or a bad mother. Like the other 10-20 percent of all childbearing women who have a postpartum reaction, you're struggling with the tremendous physical, emotional, and relationship changes that accompany childbirth. All women must struggle to some degree after having a baby. How easy or hard your adjustment is depends on how these three factors combine in your particular situation.

If you have begun practicing some of the suggestions in this book, we congratulate you. As you may have discovered, there are lots of things you can do to speed your postpartum recovery. Following the recommendations in this book can help you feel better than ever, even if you're fully recovered from a postpartum episode, or you had an easy adjustment. Learning to be more forgiving and accepting of yourself can go a long way at any point in your life toward maintaining your emotional health. Allowing friends and family to help and support you is an important lesson that can only enhance your sense of connection to others. Nurturing your relationship with your spouse or partner will strengthen your ability to cope well together during troubled times. If you come away from reading this book with nothing more than the knowledge that you must keep your pitcher full in order to be able to give of yourself to others, we will feel that we have succeeded in what we set out to do.

You Are Not To Blame

On your journey down the road to recovery, keep reminding yourself that you are not to blame for any problems you've had along the way. There is nothing you did that "caused" your postpartum reaction. It is no more your fault than the color of your eyes. For every woman, and with each pregnancy and birth, subtle interactions between biological, psychological, and relationship factors determine that particular individual's reaction to childbirth at that particular point in time. A negative, problematic reaction is not due to personal weakness or incompetence, any more than an easy postpartum adjustment is any indication of intelligence or moral fiber. Becoming depressed or anxious or disoriented does not mean that you are a failure either as a mom or a person. But it does require you, and those who care for you, to look closely at what is happening, to sort out your symptoms, and to take whatever steps are necessary to help you recover.

Do not compare your symptoms or recovery to those of other women. Doing so can lead to more negative feelings if you see yourself as worse off or recovering more slowly. If you are still not convinced that your problems aren't your fault, you may blame yourself for not doing as well as Jane or Debby or Kate. After all, if you were as strong as the one is, or as capable as the other, you'd be further along in your recovery. Or maybe she's a better mom or has figured out how to do things right. Stop this kind of thinking—*NOW!* The truth is, the more you beat yourself up over what is happening, the worse you will feel. There is no payoff here for self-criticism. Try to be accepting about your location in the recovery process, and to acknowledge the factors that are influencing you. Focus on your individual experience and what you need to do next. You have taken an enormous step by simply reading this book. You can feel confident that you *are* on the right track.

You Can Feel Better

Postpartum reactions are very treatable, especially with prompt and effective intervention, whether self-help techniques or seeking professional care. Picking up this book is an important step, because it says that you recognize or at least suspect, that something is not quite right. Before any change can occur, you must be willing to admit that you are having trouble. This takes a lot of courage.

If your symptoms are extreme or have lasted beyond six to eight weeks postpartum, we strongly recommend that you seek professional help. You may want to start by speaking with your obstetrician and getting his or her opinion. Your OB may want to see you for an evaluation or may refer you to a health-care provider who specializes in postpartum reactions. If you're receiving appropriate care, your symptoms should diminish within two to four weeks of beginning treatment. This does not mean that you will feel fully recovered, but you should be feeling at least a little better.

If you are not feeling any better after a month of treatment, discuss this with your health-care provider. It may be that you cannot see your improvement because of what you are going through, or because change is occurring too slowly for you to notice it from day to day. Ask your health-care provider to describe the changes that he or she has observed. If you're convinced of some improvement, stay the course. Otherwise, refer to our recommendations in Chapter 7 about finding the right health-care provider. Don't settle for someone who cannot effectively help you. Although recovery can be a slow-going process, with appropriate treatment, you will start to feel better soon.

Self-Help

There are many things you can do to promote your postpartum recovery. The first and most important resolution you can make is to be patient and loving toward yourself. Do not criticize or blame yourself for what is happening. Show as much understanding as you would toward a treasured friend. Try to be open and honest about your feelings, whatever they are. If you feel sad, angry, frightened, frustrated, or disappointed, acknowledge your losses. Embrace your grief. But go slowly. Don't push yourself to face or do too much, too soon. Trust yourself to know when you're ready to take the next step, to clear the next hurdle, or to risk another change.

It's essential to take good care of your physical health. Follow a healthy eating plan, exercise three times a week if you can, and get plenty of rest. These things are easier said than accomplished. Getting plenty of rest, for instance, may mean asking family members and friends to stand in for you while you put in earplugs and burrow under the covers. Do what you have to do, and don't be afraid to ask for all the support and help you need.

When you feel physically run down, take time to recharge. Don't push your body to its limit any more than it's being pushed already. Fatigue and physical exhaustion can quickly lead to your feeling worse.

For your emotional health, continue to call on family and friends. Having a shoulder to cry on or someone to listen sympathetically when you are feeling down is one of the essential components of recovery. You will feel less alone and vulnerable. Friends can be a reservoir of strength when you feel you have none left of your own. Letting friends and family help with household or child-care responsibilities will help restore your physical and emotional reserves. Be certain to let your helpers know what you need, and how you want things done. You can be sensitive to their feelings, but try to stay focused on what will be most helpful to you.

Trust your instincts to know what is best for you, your baby, and your immediate family.

If you develop particular symptoms, refer to the relevant pages in Chapter 4 (look at the index at the beginning of that chapter). Remind yourself that there are definite steps you can take to improve your postpartum adjustment. You are *not* helpless; you can get better. Yes, it will take some time and effort, but you can do it. Set small goals for yourself and tackle your difficulties one by one. Take breaks as you need them. Give yourself time to recharge, but do not give up. Do not treat yourself as a victim. Recovery *is* within your grasp. Always remember this.

Professional Help

If your problems require professional help, seek out a health-care provider who is supportive and sympathetic and is knowledgeable about postpartum difficulties. Finding the right person may take some persistence. You may have to speak with several health-care providers before you find the one who is right for you. It's critical to your recovery that you feel comfortable with your choice. Empower yourself by learning as much as you can about your particular postpartum difficulty, causes, and alternatives for treatment. Be certain to explore all of your options. If you don't want to pursue a particular recommendation, such as taking medicine, speak up. Ask what else can be done. What will the consequences be if you don't follow this recommendation? Can you try something else first? Make an informed decision by evaluating the answers to these questions. Become actively involved in designing your treatment plan. Do not surrender your freedom to choose what happens to you.

Recovery and Relapse

As you work on recovering from your postpartum problems, do not be discouraged if it takes time to heal. Even though postpartum reactions are very treatable, they do not go away overnight. When postpartum adjustment symptoms are intensified by more long-standing emotional issues, recovery may be slower. Whatever your circumstances, the truth is that *recovery is a process*. It is two steps forward and one step back. You may feel terrific one day because you seem so much better. Then your mood may plummet again a few days later, because that black cloud has gathered over you again. It's not your fault—this is simply the nature of recovery. Over time, your relapses will be less frequent, shorter-lived, and less intense. For now, pace your recovery. Give yourself time to heal. Remain flexible enough to make changes in your recovery plan as your needs evolve.

Use your relapses as a learning experience if you can. Think about what may have led up to the increase in trouble again, and what you might do differently next time to diminish or prevent another relapse.

Many women in the throes of a postpartum reaction are strongly committed to practicing their relaxation, taking breaks, and keeping their expectations modest. But once they start feeling better, there is a tendency to stop taking care of themselves and keeping their pitcher full, because they think they don't need to anymore. When this happens, a relapse can come as a horrible and crushing surprise. If this or something similar happens to you, do not beat yourself up for what you have done. Just turn yourself in the right direction again, and learn from your mistakes. Recognize the importance of continuing to take good care of yourself even when you're feeling well. Use your relapse as an opportunity to think ahead, as a way to troubleshoot into the future. Treated in this way, a relapse can actually improve rather than diminish your chances for a full and quick recovery.

Planning Ahead

Although the recommendations in this book are addressed specifically to postpartum adjustment, many of them will continue to enhance the quality of your life as your child grows. Taking better care of yourself physically and emotionally will give you more energy and enthusiasm. The better you feel, the more you will have to give.

If you are considering another pregnancy, or if you are pregnant now, pay special attention to Chapter 9. Designing a plan for your postpartum adjustment during your pregnancy is your best strategy for preventing another postpartum reaction. Although some postpartum reactions may recur no matter what you do, there are other problems that can be prevented, and most can be stopped from getting out of hand. With sound prenatal planning, and prompt and appropriate postpartum intervention, you will not need to suffer again as you did in the past. Things can be different the second or third time around. Give yourself a fighting chance.

Motherhood Reviewed

As you work through this process of feeling better, remind yourself of the need to reconceptualize motherhood. Being a parent is not a Hallmark card. It's not all sunshine and flowers and little hearts. It's just plain hard work much of the time, with many wonderful moments sprinkled in to keep you going. Bear this in mind, and you may feel better. Expect to have some bad days and some negative feelings. Don't expect to always feel confident and doubt-free. You are tackling one of the most important, influential jobs you will ever have. Accept that it is a difficult job, with the rewards often obscured by the daily muck and mire. It may be hard to find people to tell you that you are doing a good job. But you can tell yourself that you are, and ask your partner, family and friends, and pediatrician to tell you so, too. If you have doubts about your abilities, you can educate yourself and get reassurance that way. Take a parenting class, or check out a library book to learn about child development or child care. Look at how your baby is growing and thriving, and notice how important you are to that little life. Your baby knows that you are "Mom." That in itself is proof that you're succeeding.

Expect parenting to be tough and full of challenges. Know that the prizes for a job well done may be small and subtle—but they're there if you remember to look for them! You can be certain that "This is how it's supposed to be," rather than thinking that there's something wrong with you because "It wasn't supposed to be like this." With realistic expectations of motherhood, you can feel satisfied, confident, and proud of your accomplishments in meeting this most difficult challenge.

Resources

Resources for Self-Help Groups and Professional Referrals Postpartum

Depression After Delivery—National
P.O. Box 1282
Morrisville, PA 19067
(215)295-3994
(800)944-4PPD

Postpartum Support International
927 N. Kellogg Ave.
Santa Barbara, CA 93111
(805)967-7636

The Marcé Society (an international association of health professionals dedicated to the issues of mental health and childbearing)
c/o Michael O'Hara, Ph.D.
Department of Psychology
University of Iowa
Iowa City, IA 52242
(319)355-2452

Postpartum Adjustment Support Services (PASS-CAN)
P.O. Box 7282
Oakville, Ontario L6J 6C6 Canada
(905) 844-9009

Health and Breastfeeding Issues

La Leche League
(800)LaLeche or (708)455-7730 M-F 8 a.m. to 3 p.m. Central Time

National Institute of Mental Health Hotline About Panic (information and referral to support groups and/or professionals)
(800)64-PANIC

Resolve, Inc.—National
1310 Broadway
Somerville, MA 02144-1731
(617)623-0744
(800)558-7046

Family Resource Coalition (parent education and support)
200 S. Michigan Ave., Suite 1520
Chicago, IL 60604
(312)341-0900

Anxiety Disorders Association of America (support groups/information about anxiety)
6000 Executive Blvd.
Rockville, MD 20852-3801
(301)231-9350

National Anxiety Foundation (professional referral/information about anxiety)
3135 Custer Drive
Lexington, KY 40517-4001
(800)755-1576

Parents as Teachers National Center, Inc.
9374 Olive Boulevard
St. Louis, MO 63132
(314)432-4330

The following three resources provide comprehensive educational materials concerning women's health issues, particularly those related to reproductive function. All the organizations can also connect you with pharmaceutical sources for obtaining natural progesterone and estrogen.

Madison Pharmacy Associates (postpartum, premenstrual, menopause therapy, infertility, and endometriosis)
P.O. Box 9326
Madison, WI 53715
(800)558-7046

Women's Health Connection (similar to Madison Pharmacy Associates)
P.O. Box 6338
Madison, WI 53716-0338
(800)366-6632

Women's Health America (all Female health concerns)
P.O. Box 9690
Madison, WI 53715
(608)833-9102

A Selected List of Medical Professionals Involved in Relevant Research

Lee Cohen, M.D
Assistant Professor of Psychiatry
Harvard Medical School
Director, Perinatal Psychiatry Clinical Research Program
Clinical Psychopharmacology Unit
Department of Psychiatry
Massachusetts General Hospital
Boston, MA 02114
(617)969-3396
Use of medication during pregnancy and breastfeeding

James Hamilton, M.D.
2643 Union Street
San Francisco, CA 94123
(415)922-8833
Postpartum psychiatric syndromes—treatment options, legal issues

M.E. Ted Quigley, M.D.
Clinical Associate Professor
University of California—San Diego
9339 Genessee Avenue, Suite 200
San Diego, CA 92121
(619)455-7520
Hormonal intervention for postpartum difficulties

Deborah Sichel, M.D.
Assistant Professor of Psychiatry
Harvard Medical School
Clinical Associate, Perinatal Psychiatry Clinical Research Program
Clinical Psychopharmacology Unit
Department of Psychiatry
Massachusetts General Hospital

Boston, MA 02114
(617)969-3396
Hormonal intervention and use of medication during pregnancy and breast-feeding

Katherine L. Wisner, M.D., M.S.
Director of Women's Services
Mood Disorders Program
Case Western Reserve University
11400 Euclid Ave., Suite 200
Cleveland, OH 44106
(216) 721-4600
Use of medication during breastfeeding

Women's Stories of New Parenthood

Barrett, Nina (1994) *The Playgroup.* New York: Simon and Schuster.

Barrett, Nina (1990) *I Wish Someone Had Told Me.* New York: Simon and Schuster.

Burck, Frances Wells (1986) *Mothers Talking: Sharing the Secret.* New York: St. Martin's Press.

Chesler, Phyllis (1979) *With Child: A Diary of Motherhood.* New York: Thomas Y. Crowell, Publishers.

Galinsky, Ellen (1981) *The Six Stages of Parenthood.* Reading, MA: Addison-Wesley Publishing Co.

Gansberg, Judith, and Arthur P. Mostel (1984) *The Second Nine Months.* New York: Pocket Books.

Israeloff, Roberta (1984) *Coming to Terms.* New York: Alfred A. Knopf.

Lazarre, Jane (1986) *The Mother Knot.* Boston: Beacon Press.

Lim, Robin (1991) *Stories After the Baby's Birth: A Woman's Way to Wellness.* Berkeley, CA: Celestial Arts Press.

Matthews, Sanford J., and Maryann Bucknum Brinley (1982) *The Motherhood Survival Manual.* New York: Zebra Books.

Reynolds, Marilyn (1993) *Detour for Emmy.* Bueno Park, CA: Morning Glory Press (about teen pregnancy).

Books on Adjustment to New Parenthood (for couples)

Belsky, Jay, and John Kelly (1994) *The Transition to Parenthood: How a First Child Changes a Marriage.* New York: Delacorte Press.

Hotchner, Tracy (1988) *Childbirth and Marriage: The Transition to Parenthood.* New York: Avon Books.

Kanter, Carol N. (1983) *And Baby Makes Three: Your Feelings and Needs as New Parents.* Minneapolis: Winston Press.

Squire, Susan (1994) *For Better, For Worse: A Candid Chronicle of Couples Adjusting to Parenthood.* New York: Bantam Books.

Books on Postpartum Depression and Adjustment

Arthur, Shirley (1991) *Surviving Teen Pregnancy: Your Choices, Dreams, and Decisions.* Bueno Park, CA: Morning Glory Press.

Comport, Maggie (1990) *Surviving Motherhood: Coping With Postnatal Depression.* Bath, England: Ashgrove Press.

Dalton, Katharina (1980) *Depression After Childbirth.* Oxford, England: Oxford University Press.

Delliquadri, Lyn, and Kati Breckenridge (1978) *Mother Care.* New York: Pocket Books.

Dix, Carol (1985) *The New Mother Syndrome: Coping With Postpartum Stress and Depression.* Garden City, New York: Doubleday, Inc.

Eagan, Andrea Boroff (1985) *The Newborn Mother: Stages of Her Growth.* Boston: Little, Brown, & Co.

Eheart, Brenda Krause, and Susan Karol Martel (1983) *The Fourth Trimester: On Becoming a Mother.* Norwalk, CT: Appleton-Century Crofts.

Hamilton, James, and Patricia Harbinger, eds. (1992) *Postpartum Psychiatric Illness: A Picture Puzzle.* Philadelphia: University of Pennsylvania Press.

Kumar, R., and I. F. Brockington, eds. (1988) *Motherhood and Mental Illness: Causes and Consequences.* London: Wright Publishers.

Lewis, Cynthia Copeland (1989) *Mother's First Year.* New York: Berkley Books.

Lindsey, Jeanne Warren, and Jean Brunelli (1991) *Teens Parenting—Your Pregnant and Newborn Journey.* Beuno Park, CA: Morning Glory Press.

McBride, Angela (1973) *The Growth and Development of Mothers.* New York: Harper & Row.

Pacific Postpartum Support Society (1987) *Postpartum Depression and Anxiety: A Self-Help Guide for Mothers.* Vancouver, BC: Grandview Printing Co. Ltd.

Sapsted, Anne Marie (1990) *Banish the Post-Baby Blues.* Northamptonshire, England: Thorsons Publishing Group.

Stern, Ellen Sue (1986) *Expecting Change: The Emotional Journey Through Pregnancy.* New York: Poseidon Press.

Books on Related Health Issues

Anderson, Joan (1990) *The Single Mother's Book.* Atlanta: Peachtree Publishers.

Black, Claudia (1985) *Repeat After Me.* Denver: M.A.C. Printing and Publications.

Bourne, Edmund J. (1990) *The Anxiety and Phobia Workbook.* Oakland, CA: New Harbinger Publications.

Brazelton, T. Berry (1983) *Infants and Mothers.* New York: Delacorte Press.

Burns, David (1990) *The Feeling Good Handbook.* New York: Plume.

Catalano, Ellen, Charles Morin, James Walsh, and Wilse Webb (1990) *Getting to Sleep: Simple Effective Methods for Falling and Staying Asleep, Getting the Rest You Need, and Awakening Refreshed and Renewed.* Oakland, CA: New Harbinger Publications.

Dalton, Katharina (1990) *Once a Month.* Alameda, CA: Hunter House Publications.

Daniels, Pamela, and Kathy Weingarten (1982) *Sooner or Later: The Timing of Parenthood in Adult Lives.* New York: W.W. Norton and Co.

Davis, Martha, Elizabeth Robbins Eshelman, and Matthew McKay (1988) *The Relaxation and Stress Reduction Workbook.* Oakland, CA: New Harbinger Publications.

Foa, Edna B., and Reid Wilson (1991) *Stop Obsessing: How To Overcome Your Obsessions and Compulsions.* New York: Bantam Books.

Ford, Gillian (1992) *What's Wrong with My Hormones?* Newcastle, California: Desmond Ford Publications.

Greenspan, Miriam (1983) *A New Approach to Women and Therapy.* New York: McGraw Hill Book Co.

Huggins, Kathleen (1990) *The Nursing Mother's Companion.* Boston: The Harvard Common Press.

Johnston, Joni (1994) *Appearance Obsession: Learning To Love the Way You Look.* Deerfield Beach, FL: Health Communications, Inc.

Kirkman, Rick, and Jerry Scott (1991) *Baby Blues: This Is Going To Be Tougher Than We Thought.* Chicago: Contemporary Books, Inc.

Martorano, Joseph, and Maureen Morgan (1993) *Unmasking PMS: The Complete PMS Medical Treatment Plan.* New York: M. Evans and Co.

McGrath, Ellen (1992) *When Feeling Bad Is Good.* New York: Henry Holt and Co.

McKay, Matthew, Martha Davis, and Patrick Fanning (1983) *Messages: The Communication Skills Book.* Oakland, CA: New Harbinger Publications

McKay, Matthew, Peter D. Rogers, and Judith McKay (1989) *When Anger Hurts: Quieting the Storm Within.* Oakland, CA: New Harbinger Publications

Physician's Desk Reference, 48th Edition (1994) Montvale, NJ: Medical Economics Data Production Co.

Preston, John, and James Johnson (1993) *Clinical Psychopharmacology Made Ridiculously Simple.* Miami: MedMaster, Inc.

Preston, John D., John O'Neal, and Mary Talaga (1994) *Handbook of Clinical Psychopharmacology for Therapists.* Oakland, CA: New Harbinger Publications.

Rydman, Edward (1989) *Finding the Right Counselor for You.* Dallas: Taylor Publishing.

Taeuber, Cynthia (ed.) (1991) *Statistical Handbook on Women in America.* Phoenix: Oryx Press.

Wilson, R. Reid (1986) *Don't Panic: Taking Control of Anxiety Attacks.* New York: Harper Perennial.

Books for Fathers and Fathers-To-Be

Atalia, Bill. M. (1992) *The Thirteen Months of Pregnancy: A Guide for the Pregnant Father.* Saint Helena, California: Oddly Enough Publishers.

Epstein, Rick (1992) *Rookie Dad: Meditations from the Backyard.* New York: Hyperion Books.

Greenburg, Dan. (1986) *Confessions of a Pregnant Father.* New York: Ballantine Books.

Greenberg, Martin (1985) *The Birth of a Father.* New York: Avon Books.

Greene, Bob (1985) *Good Morning, Merry Sunshine: A Father's Journal of His Child's First Year.* New York: Penguin Books.

Shapiro, Jerrold Lee (1987) *When Men Are Pregnant: Needs and Concerns of Expectant Fathers.* New York: Delta Books.

Recommended Books on Child Care and Coping With High-Need Babies

Brazelton, T. Berry (1984) *To Listen to a Child: Understanding the Normal Problems of Growing Up.* Reading, MA: Addison-Wesley Publishing Co.

Ferber, Richard (1985) *Solving Your Child's Sleep Problem.* New York: Simon and Schuster.

Kutner, Lawrence (1993) *Pregnancy and Your Baby's First Year.* New York: Avon Books.

Lansky, Vicki, ed. (1993) *Games Babies Play: From Birth to Twelve Months.* Deephaven, MN: The Book Peddlers.

Lansky, Vicki (1985) *Getting Your Baby to Sleep (and Back to Sleep).* New York: Bantam Books.

Lansky, Vicki (1982) *Practical Parenting Tips.* Deephaven, MN: Meadowbrook Press.

Munger, Evelyn M., and Susan J. Bowdon (1993) *The New Beyond Peek-a-boo and Pat-a-cake: Activities for Baby's First Twenty-Four Months.* Piscataway, NJ: New Century Publishers.

Sammons, William A. H. (1989) *The Self-Calmed Baby.* Boston: Little, Brown & Co.

Sears, William (1987) *Nighttime Parenting: How To Get Your Baby and Child To Sleep.* New York: Penguin Books USA.

Sears, William (1985) *The Fussy Baby: How To Bring Out the Best in Your High-Need Child.* New York: Penguin Books USA.

Turecki, Stanley (1989) *The Difficult Child.* New York: Bantam Books.

Helping Professionals—Types and Sources

Psychiatrists

Psychiatrists are physicians (M.D. or D.O.) who have completed additional training in mental health issues. Many psychiatrists see medication as the first option of treatment, and may put less emphasis on "talking" therapy. Their professional association is the

American Psychiatric Association
1400 K Street NW
Washington, D.C. 20005
(202) 682-6000

Psychologists

In most states, psychologists are required to have a doctoral degree and to pass a standardized exam for licensure. Some states license master's level psychologists. Clinical and counseling psychologists have special training in psychotherapy, but are not able to administer medication. Many psychologists, however, work in close consultation with a psychiatrist who can recommend and write prescriptions for medications. The national professional association is the

American Psychological Association
750 First Street, NE
Washington, D.C. 20002-4242
(800) 374-2721

Other Therapists and Counselors

Many helping professionals have a master's degree in social work (M.S.W.) or a master's degree in marriage and family counseling (M.S. or M.A.). Many states require clinical social workers to be licensed; you will want to investigate the professional requirements in your state. Some of these therapists have considerable training and experience, but, like psychologists, they are not able to prescribe medication. Be sure to inquire whether a particular therapist works in consultation with an M.D. who can prescribe medication if needed.

There is a wide range of training backgrounds and credentials among persons who call themselves therapists or counselors. States increasingly require licensure for counselors, usually with a minimum of a master's degree in counseling, education, psychology, or a related field. Marriage and family counselors have training primarily in relationship, rather than individual issues. Pastoral counselors often place special emphasis on religious issues in therapy, and may be ordained clergypersons as well.

American Association for Marriage and Family Therapy
1100 Seventeenth Street NW, Tenth Floor
Washington, D.C. 20036-4601
(800) 374-2638

American Association of Pastoral Counselors
9504A Lee Highway
Fairfax, VA 22031
(703) 385-6967

National Association of Social Workers
750 First Street NE, Suite 700
Washington, D.C. 20002
(800) 638-8799

Other New Harbinger Self-Help Titles

Coping With Schizophrenia: A Guide For Families, $13.95
Visualization for Change, Second Edition, $13.95
Postpartum Survival Guide, $13.95
Angry All The Time: An Emergency Guide to Anger Control, $12.95
Couple Skills: Making Your Relationship Work, $12.95
Handbook of Clinical Psychopharmacology for Therapists, $39.95
The Warrior's Journey Home: Healing Men, Healing the Planet, $12.95
Weight Loss Through Persistence, $12.95
Post-Traumatic Stress Disorder: A Complete Treatment Guide, $39.95
Stepfamily Realities: How to Overcome Difficulties and Have a Happy Family, $11.95
Leaving the Fold: A Guide for Former Fundamentalists and Others Leaving Their Religion, $13.95
Father-Son Healing: An Adult Son's Guide, $12.95
The Chemotherapy Survival Guide, $11.95
Your Family/Your Self: How to Analyze Your Family System, $12.95
Being a Man: A Guide to the New Masculinity, $12.95
The Deadly Diet, Second Edition: Recovering from Anorexia & Bulimia, $11.95
Last Touch: Preparing for a Parent's Death, $11.95
Consuming Passions: Help for Compulsive Shoppers, $11.95
Self-Esteem, Second Edition, $12.95
Depression & Anxiety Mangement: An audio tape for managing emotional problems, $11.95
I Can't Get Over It, A Handbook for Trauma Survivors, $13.95
Concerned Intervention, When Your Loved One Won't Quit Alcohol or Drugs, $11.95
Redefining Mr. Right, $11.95
Dying of Embarrassment: Help for Social Anxiety and Social Phobia, $11.95
The Depression Workbook: Living With Depression and Manic Depression, $14.95
Risk-Taking for Personal Growth: A Step-by-Step Workbook, $11.95
The Marriage Bed: Renewing Love, Friendship, Trust, and Romance, $11.95
Focal Group Psychotherapy: For Mental Health Professionals, $44.95
Hot Water Therapy: Save Your Back, Neck & Shoulders in 10 Minutes a Day $11.95
Older & Wiser: A Workbook for Coping With Aging, $12.95
Prisoners of Belief: Exposing & Changing Beliefs that Control Your Life, $10.95
Be Sick Well: A Healthy Approach to Chronic Illness, $11.95
Men & Grief: A Guide for Men Surviving the Death of a Loved One., $12.95
When the Bough Breaks: A Helping Guide for Parents of Sexually Abused Childern, $11.95
Love Addiction: A Guide to Emotional Independence, $12.95
When Once Is Not Enough: Help for Obsessive Compulsives, $11.95
The New Three Minute Meditator, $12.95
Getting to Sleep, $10.95
The Relaxation & Stress Reduction Workbook, 3rd Edition, $14.95
Leader's Guide to the Relaxation & Stress Reduction Workbook, $19.95
Beyond Grief: A Guide for Recovering from the Death of a Loved One, $10.95
Thoughts & Feelings: The Art of Cognitive Stress Intervention, $13.95
Messages: The Communication Skills Book, $12.95
The Divorce Book, $11.95
Hypnosis for Change: A Manual of Proven Techniques, 2nd Edition, $12.95
The Chronic Pain Control Workbook, $13.95
Visualization for Change, $12.95
My Parent's Keeper: Adult Children of the Emotionally Disturbed, $11.95
When Anger Hurts, $13.95
Free of the Shadows: Recovering from Sexual Violence, $12.95
Lifetime Weight Control, $11.95
The Anxiety & Phobia Workbook, $14.95
Love and Renewal: A Couple's Guide to Commitment, $12.95
The Habit Control Workbook, $12.95

Call **toll free, 1-800-748-6273**, to order. Have your Visa or Mastercard number ready. Or send a check for the titles you want to New Harbinger Publications, Inc., 5674 Shattuck Avenue, Oakland, CA 94609. Include $3.80 for the first book and 75¢ for each additional book, to cover shipping and handling. (California residents please include appropriate sales tax.) Allow four to six weeks for delivery.

Prices subject to change without notice.